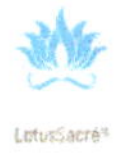

I0704324

The mistreatment of our elders

Testimonies and Revelations of a Global Scourge

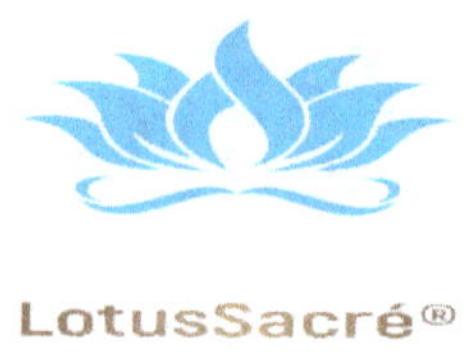

LotusSacré®

COPYRIGHT © 2024 LOTUSSACRÉ®

All rights reserved. No part of this book may be reproduced, distributed, or transmitted in any form or by any means, including photocopying, recording, or other electronic or mechanical methods, without the prior written permission of the author, except in the case of brief quotations embodied in critical reviews and certain other noncommercial uses permitted by copyright law. For permission requests, please contact the author at alizeesa@gmail.com

First Edition September 2024

This is a work of non-fiction. Any references to historical events, real people, or real places are used factually. All other names, characters, places, and incidents are the product of the author's research and imagination. Any resemblance to actual events, places, or persons, living or dead, is entirely coincidental.

TABLE OF CONTENTS

INTRODUCTION

In recent years, a disturbing reality has come to light, shaking the foundations of our society's care for its most vulnerable members. The abuse of our elders in retirement homes, once a whispered concern, has emerged as a global scourge that demands our immediate attention and action. This book seeks to shed light on this pervasive issue, bringing together testimonies, revelations, and in-depth analysis to understand the failures of our societies in protecting those who have given us so much.

The Importance of Addressing Elder Abuse

As our global population ages, the care and well-being of older adults have become critical concerns. Retirement homes, designed to provide comfort, safety, and dignified living for our elders, have unfortunately become sites of unimaginable suffering for many. The abuse that occurs

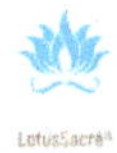
LotusSacré

within these institutions is not just a violation of human rights; it's a betrayal of the trust placed in our care systems and a reflection of deeper societal issues.

The importance of addressing elder abuse cannot be overstated. It affects not only the direct victims but also their families, caregivers, and the very fabric of our communities. By ignoring or minimizing this issue, we risk perpetuating a cycle of neglect and indifference that threatens the dignity and well-being of our future selves.

Objectives of the Book

This book aims to:

1. Expose the reality of elder abuse in retirement homes across the globe.
2. Analyze the contributing factors that allow such abuse to persist.
3. Explore the various forms of abuse, from physical and psychological to financial and neglectful.

4. Examine the role of artificial intelligence in detecting and preventing elder abuse.
5. Provide a platform for victims and their families to share their stories.
6. Investigate successful initiatives and reforms from different countries.
7. Offer practical solutions and recommendations for prevention and intervention.
8. Inspire action among readers, policymakers, and care providers to combat this issue.

Research Methodology

To ensure a comprehensive and accurate portrayal of elder abuse in retirement homes, this book employs a multi-faceted research approach:

1. **Literature Review**: An extensive review of academic studies, government reports, and journalistic investigations provides the foundation for our understanding of the issue.

2. **Data Analysis**: Statistical data from various countries and international organizations have been analyzed to present a global perspective on the prevalence and patterns of elder abuse.

3. **Expert Interviews**: Conversations with gerontologists, elder care professionals, policymakers, and legal experts offer insights into the complexities of the problem and potential solutions.

4. **Case Studies**: Detailed examinations of specific incidents and institutions provide concrete examples of abuse and its consequences.

5. **Testimonials**: First-hand accounts from victims, their families, and whistleblowers bring a human face to the statistics and analysis.

6. **AI Integration**: Exploration of how artificial intelligence is being used to detect and prevent elder abuse, including analysis of AI-generated data and case studies of AI implementation in care settings.

As we embark to uncover the truth about elder abuse in retirement homes, it is crucial to approach the subject with both sensitivity and determination. The stories and information contained within these pages may be difficult to confront, but they are essential to understanding and addressing this critical issue.

By the end of this book, readers will not only have a comprehensive understanding of the problem but also be equipped with the knowledge and motivation to take action. Whether you are a family member concerned about a loved one, a professional in the elder care industry, a policymaker, or simply a concerned citizen, this book calls on you to join the fight against elder abuse and work towards a future where our elders receive the care, respect, and dignity they deserve.

LotusSacré®

CHAPTER 1

HISTORY OF RETIREMENT HOMES

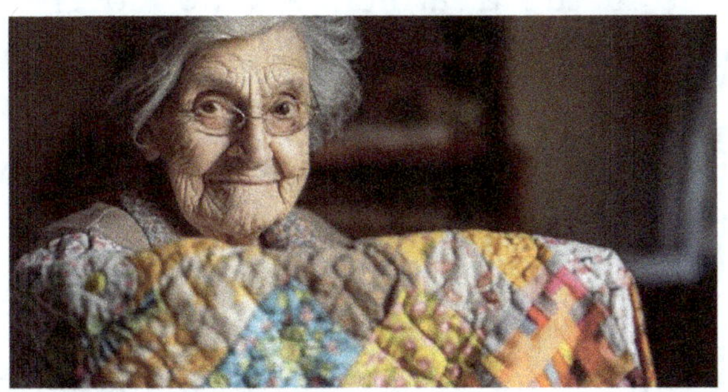

The concept of retirement homes, as we know them today, is the result of centuries of social, economic, and cultural evolution. To fully understand the current state of elder care and the challenges we face in combating abuse in these institutions, we must first examine their historical roots and development. This chapter will take you on a journey through time, tracing the evolution of retirement homes from their earliest incarnations to the modern establishments we see today.

Our focus will be primarily on France, a country with a rich history in social welfare and elder care. France's experience provides a compelling case study that reflects broader European and Western trends in the treatment of the elderly. By understanding this history, we gain invaluable insights into how societal attitudes towards aging have shifted over time, and how these changes have shaped our current elder care systems.

We will explore the transformation from medieval hospices run by religious orders to the state-regulated Établissements d'Hébergement pour Personnes Âgées Dépendantes (EHPADs) of today. This journey will reveal not just changes in physical infrastructure, but also evolving philosophies of care, the growing involvement of the state in elder welfare, and the increasing recognition of the unique needs of aging populations.

Additionally, this chapter will provide an overview of the different types of retirement homes that exist in France

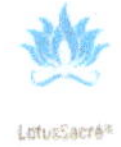

today. Each type of establishment caters to different levels of independence and care needs, reflecting the diverse requirements of the elderly population. Understanding these distinctions is crucial for comprehending the landscape of elder care and the specific contexts in which abuse can occur.

Finally, we will delve into the role and mission of EHPADs, the most common form of retirement home in France today. By examining their intended functions and responsibilities, we lay the groundwork for later discussions on how and why these institutions sometimes fail in their duties, leading to the abuse and neglect that this book aims to expose and address.

As we embark on this historical journey, it's important to remember that the story of retirement homes is not just about buildings and institutions. It's a narrative about how society values and cares for its elderly members. By understanding this history, we can better appreciate the progress that has been made, recognize the

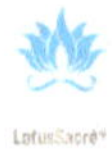

challenges that persist, and envision a future where dignity in old age is not just an ideal, but a reality for all.

Evolution of Retirement Homes in France

The history of retirement homes in France is a testament to the country's changing approach to elder care over the centuries. This evolution can be traced through several key periods:

1. Medieval Era: The Rise of Hospices

In medieval France, the care of the elderly was primarily a family responsibility. However, for those without family support, religious institutions stepped in. Monasteries and convents often provided shelter and care for the elderly poor, establishing what we might consider the earliest forms of retirement homes. These hospices, while offering basic care, were often overcrowded and focused more on spiritual comfort than physical well-being.

The concept of the hospice originated from Christian traditions of charity and hospitality. These institutions, often run by monastic orders, provided a place for the sick, the poor, and the elderly who had nowhere else to go. While they offered shelter and basic sustenance, the quality of care was often rudimentary by modern standards. The focus was primarily on providing for spiritual needs, with physical comfort being a secondary concern.

It's important to note that these early hospices were not exclusive to the elderly. They housed a mix of society's most vulnerable - the sick, the poor, orphans, and the aged. This lack of specialization meant that the specific needs of the elderly were often overlooked or inadequately addressed.

Despite their limitations, these medieval hospices represented the first systematic attempt to provide institutional care for the elderly outside the family structure. They laid the groundwork for the more

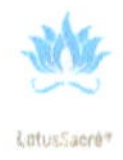

specialized care institutions that would develop in later centuries.

2. 17th-18th Centuries: The Hôpital Général

The 17th century marked a significant shift in the approach to social welfare in France, including elder care. In 1656, Louis XIV established the Hôpital Général in Paris, an institution that would have a profound impact on the care of the elderly and other vulnerable populations.

The Hôpital Général was not a medical facility in the modern sense, but rather a vast complex of buildings designed to house the poor, including many elderly individuals who could not support themselves. This development represented a move towards greater state involvement in social welfare, shifting some of the responsibility for care from religious institutions to the government.

However, the conditions in the Hôpital Général were often harsh. The institution

was as much about controlling and containing poverty as it was about providing care. Residents, including the elderly, were often subjected to strict regimes of work and prayer. The focus was on moral reform rather than comfort or specialized care for the aged.

Despite its shortcomings, the establishment of the Hôpital Général was a crucial step in the evolution of elder care. It set a precedent for state involvement in the welfare of the elderly and other vulnerable populations, a principle that would continue to develop in the centuries to come.

3. 19th Century: The Hospices Civils

The 19th century saw further developments in the institutionalization of elder care in France with the establishment of the Hospices Civils in many French cities. These institutions were more specifically focused on caring for the elderly poor, representing a step towards more specialized elder care.

The Hospices Civils were typically run by local authorities rather than religious orders, reflecting the continuing shift towards secular, state-managed care. They provided basic accommodation, food, and some level of medical care for elderly individuals who could not be supported by their families or communities.

However, these institutions still faced significant challenges. They were often overcrowded and underfunded, struggling to meet the needs of a growing elderly population. The care provided was basic, focusing on shelter and sustenance rather than comprehensive medical or psychological support.

Despite these limitations, the Hospices Civils represented an important step in the evolution of elder care. They recognized the elderly as a distinct group with specific needs, setting the stage for more specialized care in the future.

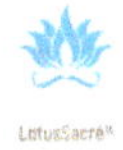

4. Early 20th Century: The Emergence of Maisons de Retraite

The early 20th century marked a significant shift in the approach to elder care in France with the emergence of "maisons de retraite" or retirement homes as we more closely recognize them today. This development reflected growing awareness of the specific needs of the elderly population and a move towards more specialized care.

Unlike their predecessors, maisons de retraite were designed specifically for older adults. They began to focus not just on providing basic shelter and sustenance, but also on addressing the social and recreational needs of residents. This shift represented an important step towards recognizing the dignity and quality of life of elderly individuals.

However, it's crucial to note that these early retirement homes were still primarily seen as a last resort. They were typically used by those who could not be cared for by their families, either due to lack of resources or

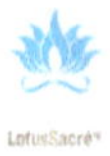

the absence of family members. The stigma associated with "sending away" elderly relatives meant that many families only turned to these institutions when they had no other options.

Despite these limitations, the emergence of maisons de retraite signaled an important shift in societal attitudes towards aging and elder care. It laid the groundwork for more comprehensive and specialized care models that would develop in the latter half of the century.

5. Post-World War II: Modernization and Expansion

The period following World War II brought about significant changes in French society that had profound impacts on elder care. Several factors contributed to a rapid expansion and modernization of retirement homes during this time:

1. **Demographic Shifts**: The post-war period saw a dramatic increase in life

expectancy, resulting in a larger elderly population requiring care.

2. **Changing Family Structures**: Urbanization and changes in family dynamics meant that fewer elderly individuals could rely on family members for care.

3. **Economic Growth**: The post-war economic boom provided resources for expanding and improving social services, including elder care.

4. **Government Involvement**: The French government took a more active role in regulating and funding retirement homes, recognizing elder care as a crucial social issue.

During this period, there was a significant increase in the number of retirement homes across France. These new institutions were often better equipped and staffed than their predecessors, with a greater focus on providing comfortable living conditions and medical care.

The concept of retirement homes also began to evolve. While still primarily

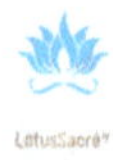

catering to those who couldn't be cared for at home, there was a growing recognition that these institutions could provide valuable services even for more independent seniors. This led to the development of a range of different types of retirement facilities catering to various levels of need and independence.

6. Late 20th Century to Present: The Rise of EHPADs

The most recent chapter in the history of French retirement homes is marked by the development of EHPADs (Établissement d'Hébergement pour Personnes Âgées Dépendantes). Established by law in 1997, EHPADs represent the most modern and comprehensive form of retirement homes in France.

EHPADs were created in response to the growing need for specialized care for dependent elderly individuals. They are designed to provide a high level of medical and personal care, alongside accommodation and social support. This

model recognizes that many elderly individuals, particularly those with chronic health conditions or cognitive impairments, require more intensive support than traditional retirement homes could provide.

Key features of EHPADs include:

1. **Medical Staff**: EHPADs are required to have medical professionals, including nurses and often a coordinating doctor, on staff.
2. **Personalized Care Plans**: Each resident has an individualized care plan tailored to their specific needs and health conditions.
3. **Specialized Units**: Many EHPADs include specialized units for residents with conditions such as Alzheimer's disease or other forms of dementia.
4. **Regulated Standards**: EHPADs are subject to strict government regulations regarding staffing levels, care quality, and facilities.

The rise of EHPADs marks a significant evolution in the approach to elder care in

France. It represents a move towards a more medicalized model of care, recognizing the complex health needs of an aging population. However, as we will explore in later chapters, this model also brings its own challenges and potential for systemic issues.

Different Types of Establishments

Today, France offers a variety of elder care options, each catering to different levels of independence and care needs:

1. **Résidences Autonomie (formerly Foyers-logements)**: These are designed for relatively independent seniors. They offer private apartments with some communal facilities and optional services such as meals or housekeeping. Residents can live independently while having access to support if needed.

2. **EHPADs**: As discussed earlier, these cater to elderly individuals who are no longer able to live independently.

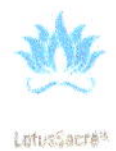

They provide comprehensive care, including medical support, personal assistance, and social activities.

3. **Résidences Services Seniors**: These are private residences offering services like meals, housekeeping, and activities, but with less medical support than EHPADs. They're often more luxurious and cater to wealthier seniors who want to maintain a high quality of life while having access to support services.

4. **Unités de Soins Longue Durée (USLD)**: These are medical facilities for elderly individuals with severe health issues requiring constant medical attention. They provide a higher level of medical care than standard EHPADs.

5. **Accueil Familial**: This involves elderly individuals being cared for in the home of an approved carer, offering a more familial environment. This option can be particularly beneficial for seniors who struggle with the institutional nature of traditional retirement homes.

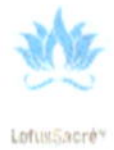

Role and Mission of EHPADs

As the primary form of residential elder care in France today, EHPADs play a crucial role in the French elder care system. Their missions include:

1. **Comprehensive Care**: EHPADs are designed to provide all-encompassing care for dependent elderly individuals. This includes not just accommodation, but also medical care, personal assistance, and social support.
2. **Medical Support**: Unlike other forms of retirement homes, EHPADs have medical staff on-site, including nurses and often a coordinating doctor. They are equipped to handle various health issues common in the elderly population.
3. **Maintaining Dignity and Independence**: Despite catering to dependent individuals, EHPADs aim to maintain residents' dignity and as much independence as possible. This involves personalized care plans and activities

designed to stimulate cognitive and physical abilities.

4. **Social Integration**: EHPADs are tasked with ensuring that residents don't become isolated. They organize social activities, outings, and encourage family visits to maintain social connections.

5. **End-of-Life Care**: Many EHPADs are equipped to provide palliative care, ensuring comfort and dignity in the final stages of life.

6. **Alzheimer's and Dementia Care**: Many EHPADs have specialized units for individuals with Alzheimer's disease or other forms of dementia, providing targeted care for these conditions.

The evolution of retirement homes in France reflects broader societal changes in attitudes towards aging, care, and the role of the state in providing for its elderly citizens. From medieval hospices to modern EHPADs, each stage in this evolution has brought both progress and new challenges.

Today's retirement homes, particularly EHPADs, represent the culmination of centuries of development in elder care. They aim to provide comprehensive, dignified care for France's aging population. However, as we will explore in subsequent chapters, the reality often falls short of these ideals.

Understanding this history is crucial as we delve into the current issues facing retirement homes, including the troubling prevalence of elder abuse. By recognizing how far we've come, we can better appreciate the progress that's been made while also critically examining where the system continues to fall short.

As we move forward, it's essential to keep in mind that the story of retirement homes is far from over. The challenges we face today will shape the next chapter in this ongoing evolution, hopefully leading to even better, more compassionate care for our elderly citizens in the future.

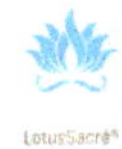

CALL TO ACTION

- Research the history of retirement homes in your local area and create a timeline to share with your community.
- Visit a local retirement home and interview long-term residents about their experiences over the years.
- Organize a community event to discuss the evolution of elder care and brainstorm future improvements.

Your Review Helps:

- Raise awareness about elder abuse in retirement homes
- Support independent authors tackling crucial social issues
- Encourage more research and action on elder care reform

How to Leave a Review:

- Go to the book's Amazon page
- Click "Write a customer review"
- Share your honest thoughts and experiences
- Click submit

If you found value in this book, please consider leaving a 5-star review!

Your support helps fuel further investigation into elder care issues and promotes positive change in our retirement homes. By sharing your thoughts, you're giving a voice to those who often go unheard and contributing to a movement for dignity and respect for our elders.

Together, we can make a difference in the lives of our seniors.

This version maintains the structure and purpose of the original text while adapting the content to fit the theme of your book on elder abuse in retirement homes. It emphasizes the importance of raising awareness about elder abuse and encourages readers to contribute to positive change through their reviews.

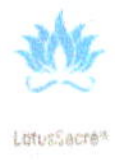

CHAPTER 2

THE SCANDALS REVEALED

In recent years, a series of shocking revelations have brought the issue of elder abuse in retirement homes to the forefront of public consciousness. These scandals, uncovered through painstaking journalistic investigations and courageous testimonies from victims and their families, have exposed a dark underbelly to the eldercare system that many had preferred to ignore.

This chapter delves into these revelations, shining a light on the systemic issues plaguing many retirement homes and long-term care facilities. We will explore how investigative journalism has played a crucial role in exposing these abuses, examine the heart-wrenching testimonies of those who have suffered, and analyze the

often inadequate responses from authorities and care home establishments.

At the heart of this chapter is a fundamental question: How could such widespread abuse occur in institutions meant to care for society's most vulnerable members? By examining these scandals in detail, we aim not only to expose the horrifying reality faced by many elderly residents but also to understand the systemic failures that allow such abuses to persist.

It's important to note that while this chapter deals with distressing content, its purpose is not to sensationalize but to inform and galvanize action. By understanding the full extent of the problem, we can begin to formulate effective solutions and work towards a future where our elderly population receives the care and respect they deserve.

LotusSacré

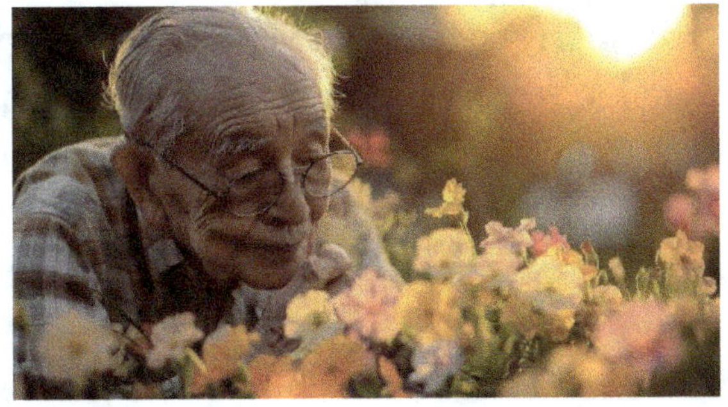

Journalistic Investigations

"Les Fossoyeurs" by Victor Castanet

One of the most significant exposés in recent years came from French journalist Victor Castanet's book "Les Fossoyeurs" (The Gravediggers), published in 2022. This groundbreaking investigation sent shockwaves through French society and beyond, revealing widespread abuse and neglect in France's largest private nursing home group, Orpea.

Castanet's three-year investigation uncovered a system where profit was prioritized over the well-being of residents. Key findings included:

1. **Rationing of Care**: The investigation revealed that essential care items, including food and hygiene products, were strictly rationed to cut costs, often leaving residents malnourished and in unsanitary conditions.

2. **Staffing Issues**: The book exposed chronic understaffing and high turnover rates, leading to inadequate care for residents.

3. **Financial Malpractices**: Castanet uncovered evidence of financial irregularities, including the misuse of public funds intended for resident care.

4. **Covering Up Deaths**: Perhaps most disturbingly, the investigation suggested that some deaths resulting from neglect were covered up or misreported.

The publication of "Les Fossoyeurs" had immediate and far-reaching consequences. It led to a sharp drop in Orpea's stock price, triggered government investigations, and sparked a national debate about the quality of elder care in France.

Other Notable Investigations

While "Les Fossoyeurs" stands out for its comprehensive nature and impact, it's far from the only journalistic investigation to uncover abuse in retirement homes. Other notable investigations include:

1. **"Maison de Retraite" Documentary (2018)**: This French television documentary used hidden cameras to expose neglect and abuse in several nursing homes across France.
2. **"Care Home Undercover" by BBC Panorama (2019)**: In the UK, this investigation revealed shocking abuse at a care home in County Durham, including staff mocking and bullying residents with dementia.
3. **"Dirty Business" by Stern Magazine (2019)**: This German investigation exposed systemic issues in private care homes, including understaffing and neglect of residents.

These investigations, along with many others, have played a crucial role in

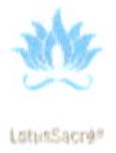

bringing the issue of elder abuse to public attention and spurring calls for reform.

Testimonies from Victims and Families

While journalistic investigations provide a broad overview of systemic issues, it's the personal testimonies of victims and their families that truly bring home the human cost of elder abuse. These stories put faces and names to the statistics, making the reality of abuse impossible to ignore.

Justina's Story

Justina, an 87-year-old resident of a nursing home in Lyon, suffered in silence for months before her daughter noticed something was wrong. "Mom always seemed anxious when we visited," her daughter recounted. "She lost weight, developed bedsores, and seemed to flinch when the staff approached her."

It was only when Justina's daughter installed a hidden camera in her room that the full extent of the abuse became clear.

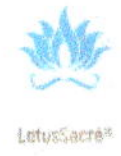

The footage showed staff roughly handling Justina, ignoring her calls for help, and leaving her in soiled clothing for hours.

The Dubois Family's Fight

The Dubois family's experience highlights the struggle many families face in getting justice for their loved ones. After their father, Pierre, died in a nursing home, they noticed suspicious bruising on his body. Despite their concerns, the home insisted these were normal signs of aging.

It took months of persistence, including hiring a private investigator and rallying other families, before the authorities took their complaints seriously. The subsequent investigation revealed a pattern of neglect and physical abuse in the home.

Anonymous Testimonies

Many victims and families choose to remain anonymous, fearing retaliation or stigma. However, their stories are no less powerful:

- *"They treated her like she wasn't even human anymore," one son said of his mother's treatment. "It was like they forgot these were people with lives and families who loved them."*
- *A former nurse speaking anonymously described the impossible conditions: "We were so understaffed, it was impossible to provide proper care. I left because I couldn't bear the guilt anymore."*

These testimonies, and countless others like them, paint a picture of a system where the dignity and well-being of the elderly are often sacrificed for convenience or profit.

Reactions from Authorities and Establishments

The revelations of abuse in retirement homes have elicited a range of responses from authorities and the establishments themselves. These reactions have varied from promises of reform to denial and attempts to downplay the issues.

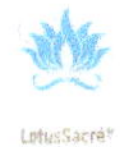

Government Response

In France, the revelations in "Les Fossoyeurs" prompted immediate government action:

1. **Investigations**: The government launched official investigations into Orpea and other major care home groups.
2. **Regulatory Changes**: Promises were made to strengthen oversight of care homes, including more frequent and thorough inspections.
3. **Funding Reviews**: The government pledged to review how public funds for elder care are allocated and monitored.

Similar patterns have been seen in other countries following major scandals, with governments often promising stricter regulations and increased funding for elder care.

Industry Reaction

The reaction from the care home industry has been mixed:

1. **Denial and Minimization**: Some establishments have attempted to downplay the extent of the problems, characterizing the exposed abuses as isolated incidents.
2. **Promises of Reform**: Many care home groups have publicly committed to improving their practices, including better staff training and more transparent reporting.
3. **Defensive Posturing**: Some industry representatives have pointed to systemic issues like underfunding and staff shortages as root causes, arguing that individual homes shouldn't bear all the blame.

Public Outcry and Civil Society Response

The scandals have also mobilized civil society:

1. **Advocacy Groups**: Elder rights organizations have used these revelations to push for stronger protections for nursing home residents.
2. **Legal Action**: In many cases, the exposés have led to class action lawsuits against care home groups.
3. **Public Awareness**: There has been a marked increase in public discourse about elder care, with many calling for a fundamental rethinking of how society cares for its aging population.

The scandals revealed through journalistic investigations and personal testimonies have laid bare the urgent need for reform in the elder care system. They have shown that abuse and neglect in retirement homes are not isolated incidents, but symptoms of deeper, systemic issues.

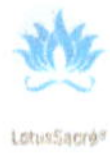

These revelations serve as a call to action. They challenge us to confront uncomfortable truths about how our society treats its most vulnerable members and to work towards creating a system where dignity, respect, and quality care are guaranteed for all elderly individuals.

As we move forward, it's crucial that we don't allow these stories to fade from public consciousness. The courage of journalists, whistleblowers, and families in bringing these abuses to light must be matched by sustained effort to enact meaningful change. Only then can we hope to create a future where our elderly population receives the care and respect they deserve.

CALL TO ACTION

- Write to your local representatives, asking what measures they're taking to prevent elder abuse in retirement homes.
- Share reputable investigative reports on social media to spread awareness about elder abuse scandals.

- Start a book club or discussion group focused on investigative journalism pieces about elder care issues.

Please Share Your Thoughts on Amazon!

Your Review Helps:

- Raise awareness about elder abuse in retirement homes
- Support independent authors tackling crucial social issues
- Encourage more research and action on elder care reform

How to Leave a Review:

- Go to the book's Amazon page
- Click "Write a customer review"
- Share your honest thoughts and experiences
- Click submit

If you found value in this book, please consider leaving a 5-star review!

Your support helps fuel further investigation into elder care issues and promotes positive change in our retirement

homes. By sharing your thoughts, you're giving a voice to those who often go unheard and contributing to a movement for dignity and respect for our elders.

Together, we can make a difference in the lives of our seniors.

This version maintains the structure and purpose of the original text while adapting the content to fit the theme of your book on elder abuse in retirement homes. It emphasizes the importance of raising awareness about elder abuse and encourages readers to contribute to positive change through their reviews.

CHAPTER 3

TYPES OF ABUSE

Elder abuse in retirement homes is a complex and multifaceted issue that manifests in various forms. Understanding these different types of abuse is crucial for identifying, preventing, and addressing mistreatment of the elderly. This chapter will delve into four main categories of abuse commonly encountered in retirement homes: physical abuse, psychological abuse, neglect and abandonment, and financial abuse.

It's important to note that these categories are not mutually exclusive. In many cases, an elderly person may experience multiple forms of abuse simultaneously, compounding the trauma and negative impact on their well-being. Additionally, what might begin as one form of abuse can

often escalate or lead to other types of mistreatment.

As we explore each type of abuse, we will:

1. Define and describe the abuse category
2. Provide examples of how it manifests in retirement home settings
3. Discuss the signs and symptoms that may indicate this type of abuse is occurring
4. Examine the potential short-term and long-term impacts on the elderly victims

By gaining a comprehensive understanding of these different forms of abuse, we can better equip ourselves to recognize warning signs, advocate for the elderly, and work towards creating safer, more dignified environments for our aging population.

LotusSacré

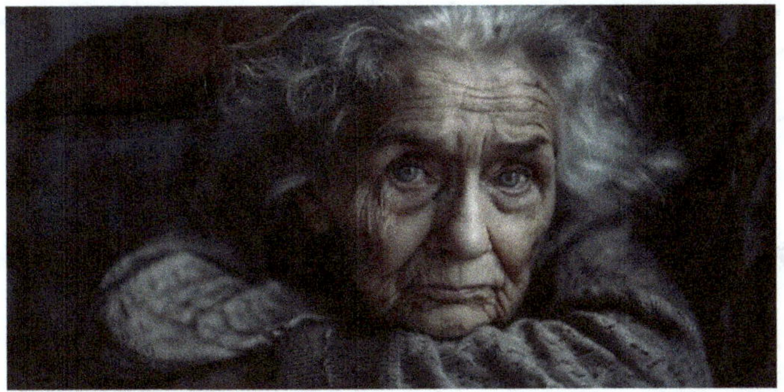

Physical Abuse

Physical abuse is perhaps the most immediately recognizable form of elder mistreatment. It involves the use of physical force that may result in bodily injury, physical pain, or impairment.

Definition and Examples

Physical abuse in retirement homes can take many forms, including but not limited to:

1. Hitting, slapping, or pushing
2. Inappropriate use of restraints (physical or chemical)
3. Force-feeding
4. Rough handling during care routines

5. Inappropriate administration of medication (over-medicating or withholding necessary medication)

Signs and Symptoms

Indicators of physical abuse may include:

1. Unexplained bruises, welts, or scars
2. Broken bones or sprains
3. Burns or abrasions
4. Signs of restraint on wrists or ankles
5. Broken eyeglasses or frames
6. Fearfulness around certain staff members
7. Sudden changes in behavior or emotional state

Impact on Victims

The effects of physical abuse can be severe and long-lasting:

1. Physical injuries and chronic pain
2. Decreased mobility and independence
3. Increased risk of future health problems
4. Psychological trauma, including depression and anxiety

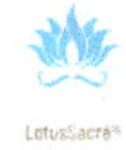

5. Increased mortality risk

Case Study: The Story of Robert

Robert, an 82-year-old resident with early-stage dementia, began showing unexplained bruises on his arms and torso. His daughter noticed he became agitated when certain staff members entered his room. An investigation revealed that an overworked and frustrated night shift worker had been roughly handling Robert during nighttime care routines. The physical abuse had exacerbated Robert's confusion and anxiety, significantly impacting his quality of life.

Psychological Abuse

Psychological or emotional abuse can be harder to detect than physical abuse but can be equally damaging to an elderly person's well-being.

Definition and Examples

Psychological abuse involves inflicting mental pain, anguish, or distress through

verbal or nonverbal acts. In retirement homes, this may include:

1. Verbal aggression, insults, or humiliation
2. Intimidation or threats
3. Isolation from friends, family, or regular activities
4. Ignoring the elderly person or giving them the "silent treatment"
5. Infantilizing behavior (treating the elderly person like a child)

Signs and Symptoms

Indicators of psychological abuse may include:

1. Unexplained or uncharacteristic changes in behavior
2. Withdrawal from social interactions
3. Depression or anxiety
4. Fearfulness or agitation
5. Loss of interest in previously enjoyed activities
6. Low self-esteem or self-worth
7. Sleep disturbances

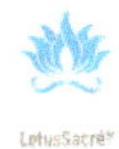

Impact on Victims

The effects of psychological abuse can be profound and long-lasting:

1. Decreased cognitive function
2. Increased risk of depression and anxiety disorders
3. Social withdrawal and isolation
4. Increased risk of physical health problems
5. Loss of self-esteem and sense of identity
6. In severe cases, increased risk of suicide

Case Study: Maria's Experience

Maria, a 75-year-old resident, became increasingly withdrawn and refused to participate in social activities. Her family noticed she seemed fearful and anxious. It was discovered that a staff member had been constantly belittling Maria, making fun of her accent, and threatening to withhold care if she complained. The psychological abuse had severely impacted Maria's mental health and quality of life.

Neglect and Abandonment

Neglect is one of the most common forms of elder abuse in retirement homes, often resulting from systemic issues such as understaffing or poor training.

Definition and Examples

Neglect involves the failure to provide for an elderly person's basic needs. This can include:

1. Failure to provide adequate food or water
2. Neglecting personal hygiene needs
3. Failure to provide necessary medication or medical care
4. Leaving a person in unsanitary or unsafe living conditions
5. Failure to prevent bedsores or attend to other medical needs

Abandonment, an extreme form of neglect, involves desertion of an elderly person by an individual who has assumed responsibility for their care.

Signs and Symptoms

Indicators of neglect or abandonment may include:

1. Malnutrition or dehydration
2. Untreated medical conditions
3. Poor personal hygiene
4. Unsanitary or unsafe living conditions
5. Unsuitable clothing for the weather
6. Bedsores or other signs of improper care
7. Signs of withdrawal or depression

Impact on Victims

The effects of neglect and abandonment can be severe:

1. Malnutrition and related health issues
2. Worsening of existing medical conditions
3. Development of new health problems
4. Increased risk of falls and injuries
5. Psychological distress, including depression and anxiety
6. In severe cases, increased mortality risk

Case Study: The Plight of James

James, an 88-year-old resident with limited mobility, developed severe bedsores and showed signs of malnutrition. Investigation revealed chronic understaffing at the facility, resulting in residents like James not receiving proper care, regular repositioning, or adequate nutrition. The neglect had severely impacted James' health and quality of life, requiring hospitalization and intensive treatment.

Financial Abuse

Financial abuse is a growing concern in retirement homes, often going hand-in-hand with other forms of abuse.

Definition and Examples

Financial abuse involves the illegal or improper use of an elderly person's funds, property, or assets. In retirement homes, this may include:

1. Theft of money or valuables

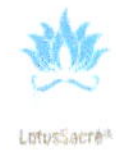
LotusSacré

2. Forging an elderly person's signature
3. Coercing or deceiving an elderly person into signing documents (e.g., contracts or wills)
4. Improper use of power of attorney
5. Charging for services not provided or overcharging for services
6. Using an elderly person's funds for staff or facility benefit without permission

Signs and Symptoms

Indicators of financial abuse may include:

1. Unexplained withdrawals from bank accounts
2. Missing personal belongings or valuables
3. Sudden changes in financial conditions
4. Unexpected changes to wills or other financial documents
5. Unpaid bills despite adequate financial resources
6. Anxiety about personal finances
7. Signatures on documents that appear forged or suspicious

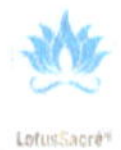

Impact on Victims

The effects of financial abuse can be devastating:

1. Loss of financial security and independence
2. Inability to afford necessary care or quality of life improvements
3. Psychological distress, including depression and anxiety
4. Increased vulnerability to other forms of abuse
5. Loss of trust in caregivers and institutions

Case Study: The Exploitation of Eleanor

Eleanor, a 79-year-old resident with mild cognitive impairment, noticed her jewelry going missing. Her son also found unusual bank withdrawals. An investigation uncovered a staff member who had been stealing from Eleanor and other residents, as well as coercing them to change their bank details. The financial abuse had not only impacted Eleanor's financial security

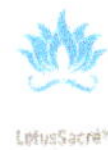

but also her trust in the care home and its staff.

Understanding these different types of abuse - physical, psychological, neglect and abandonment, and financial - is crucial in addressing the broader issue of elder abuse in retirement homes. Each form of abuse has its unique characteristics, signs, and impacts, but all share the common thread of violating the dignity, security, and well-being of elderly individuals.

It's important to remember that these types of abuse often co-occur and can exacerbate each other. For instance, an elderly person experiencing financial abuse may be more vulnerable to neglect if they can't afford proper care, or someone enduring psychological abuse may be less likely to report physical mistreatment.

Recognizing the signs of these various forms of abuse is the first step in addressing this critical issue. It empowers

family members, caregivers, and the broader community to identify potential abuse and take action. Moreover, understanding the multifaceted nature of elder abuse highlights the need for comprehensive approaches to prevention and intervention.

As we move forward, it's crucial to use this knowledge to inform policies, training programs, and support systems in retirement homes. By doing so, we can work towards creating environments where all forms of abuse are recognized, prevented, and swiftly addressed, ensuring that our elderly population receives the care, respect, and dignity they deserve.

CALL TO ACTION

- Learn to recognize the signs of different types of elder abuse and share this knowledge with friends and family.
- Volunteer at a local elder rights organization to help educate others about these issues.

- Create and distribute informational pamphlets about elder abuse in your community.

Please Share Your Thoughts on Amazon!

Your Review Helps:

- Raise awareness about elder abuse in retirement homes
- Support independent authors tackling crucial social issues
- Encourage more research and action on elder care reform

How to Leave a Review:

- Go to the book's Amazon page
- Click "Write a customer review"
- Share your honest thoughts and experiences
- Click submit

If you found value in this book, please consider leaving a 5-star review!

Your support helps fuel further investigation into elder care issues and promotes positive change in our retirement

homes. By sharing your thoughts, you're giving a voice to those who often go unheard and contributing to a movement for dignity and respect for our elders.

Together, we can make a difference in the lives of our seniors.

This version maintains the structure and purpose of the original text while adapting the content to fit the theme of your book on elder abuse in retirement homes. It emphasizes the importance of raising awareness about elder abuse and encourages readers to contribute to positive change through their reviews.

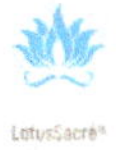

CHAPTER 4

CONTRIBUTING FACTORS

The abuse and neglect of elderly residents in retirement homes, as distressing as it is, rarely occurs in isolation. Rather, it is often the result of a complex interplay of systemic issues that create an environment where abuse can occur and persist. Understanding these contributing factors is crucial for addressing the root causes of elder abuse and developing effective prevention strategies.

In this chapter, we will discuss three primary contributing factors to elder abuse in retirement homes:

1. Lack of staff and insufficient training
2. Financial pressures and the search for profit
3. Management and supervision issues

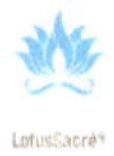

By examining these factors in depth, we can begin to understand why abuse occurs despite the best intentions of many in the eldercare industry. This understanding is crucial for developing comprehensive solutions that address not just the symptoms of abuse, but its underlying causes.

It's important to note that while these factors can contribute to an environment where abuse is more likely to occur, they do not excuse or justify abusive behavior. Rather, recognizing these systemic issues allows us to move beyond simply blaming individuals and towards creating meaningful, lasting change in the eldercare system.

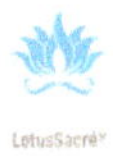
LotusSacré

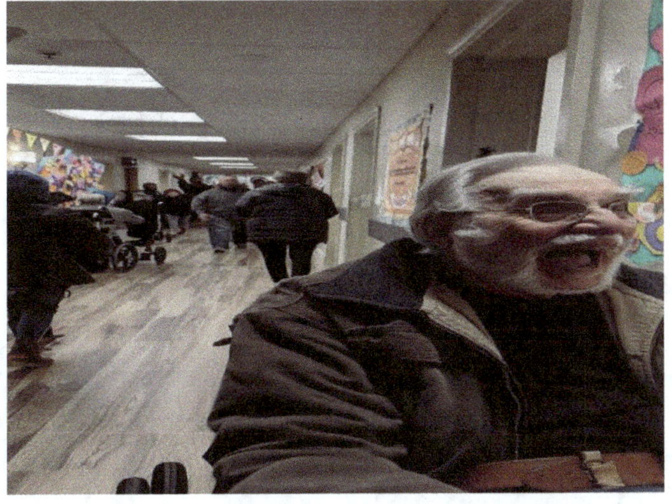

Lack of Staff and Insufficient Training

One of the most significant contributing factors to elder abuse in retirement homes is the chronic understaffing and inadequate training of caregivers. This issue has far-reaching consequences, affecting the quality of care provided and increasing the risk of abuse and neglect.

Understaffing

Understaffing in retirement homes is a pervasive problem across many countries. The reasons for this are multifaceted:

1. **High Turnover Rates**: The demanding nature of the work, coupled with often low pay and challenging working conditions, leads to high staff turnover. This creates a constant cycle of hiring and training new staff, which can be costly and time-consuming.
2. **Budget Constraints**: Many facilities, particularly those relying on public funding, operate under tight budgets that limit their ability to hire and retain adequate staff.
3. **Increasing Demand**: As populations age, the demand for eldercare services is increasing, often outpacing the growth in the caregiving workforce.
4. **Challenging Work Environment**: The physical and emotional demands of caregiving can make it difficult to attract and retain staff, particularly in a competitive job market.

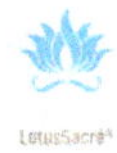

The consequences of understaffing are severe:

- **Increased Workload**: With fewer staff members, each caregiver is responsible for more residents. This can lead to rushed care, missed tasks, and increased stress for both caregivers and residents.
- **Burnout**: Overworked staff are more likely to experience burnout, which can lead to irritability, decreased empathy, and in some cases, abusive behavior.
- **Neglect**: When there aren't enough staff members to attend to all residents' needs, unintentional neglect can occur. This might involve delays in responding to calls for assistance, inadequate personal care, or overlooked medical needs.
- **Increased Risk of Errors**: Overworked and stressed staff are more likely to make mistakes, which can range from minor oversights to serious medical errors.

Case Study: The Night Shift Crisis

In a mid-sized retirement home in Ontario, Canada, chronic understaffing led to a crisis during night shifts. With only two staff members responsible for 60 residents, many of whom required regular night-time assistance, it became impossible to meet all residents' needs. This resulted in residents being left in soiled bedding, missed medication doses, and increased fall incidents as residents attempted to take care of their own needs without assistance.

Insufficient Training

Even when staffing levels are adequate, insufficient training can lead to inadvertent abuse or neglect. Key issues include:

1. **Lack of Specialized Knowledge**: Caring for elderly individuals, particularly those with complex medical conditions or cognitive impairments, requires specialized knowledge and skills. Without proper training, staff may not know how to properly handle

challenging situations or provide appropriate care.

2. **Inadequate Preparation for Emotional Challenges**: Eldercare can be emotionally taxing. Without proper training in stress management and emotional resilience, caregivers may struggle to maintain professional boundaries and appropriate behavior.

3. **Insufficient Focus on Abuse Prevention**: Many training programs fail to adequately address the issue of elder abuse, leaving staff ill-equipped to recognize and report potential abuse.

4. **Lack of Cultural Competence**: As populations become more diverse, many staff members lack training in cultural competence, leading to misunderstandings or unintentional disrespect of residents' cultural practices and beliefs.

5. **Incomplete Emergency Preparedness**: Insufficient training in emergency procedures can lead to chaos and potential harm to residents during crisis situations.

The impacts of insufficient training can be far-reaching:

- **Unintentional Abuse**: Staff who lack proper training may inadvertently cause harm while attempting to provide care, such as using improper lifting techniques or mishandling residents with cognitive impairments.
- **Failure to Recognize Abuse**: Without proper training, staff may fail to recognize signs of abuse perpetrated by others, allowing it to continue unchecked.
- **Poor Quality of Care**: Inadequately trained staff may provide substandard care, negatively impacting residents' health and quality of life.
- **Increased Stress and Burnout**: Staff who feel unprepared for their roles are more likely to experience stress and burnout, potentially leading to abusive behavior.

LotusSacré®

Case Study: The Dementia Care Gap

A retirement home in Florida, specializing in dementia care, faced a series of incidents where residents with advanced dementia were being chemically restrained due to aggressive behavior. An investigation revealed that most staff had received only basic dementia care training, leaving them ill-equipped to handle challenging behaviors without resorting to medication. This lack of specialized training had led to an overreliance on chemical restraints, negatively impacting residents' quality of life and cognitive function.

Financial Pressures and the Search for Profit

The eldercare industry, particularly in countries with privatized systems, often faces intense financial pressures. While the need to maintain financial viability is understandable, an overemphasis on profit can lead to decisions that prioritize cost-cutting over quality of care, potentially contributing to abusive or neglectful situations.

The Rise of For-Profit Care

In many countries, there has been a trend towards the privatization of eldercare, with for-profit companies playing an increasingly large role in the industry. While this can bring efficiency and innovation, it also introduces new pressures:

1. **Profit Margins**: For-profit facilities face pressure from shareholders or owners to maintain or increase profit margins, which can lead to cost-cutting measures that affect care quality.
2. **Market Competition**: In a competitive market, facilities may feel pressure to keep costs low to attract residents, potentially leading to underinvestment in staff and resources.
3. **Economies of Scale**: Large chains may prioritize standardization and efficiency over personalized care to

maximize profits across multiple facilities.

The impact of these financial pressures can manifest in various ways:

- **Understaffing**: To reduce labor costs, facilities may operate with minimal staff, increasing the risk of neglect and burnout.
- **Underinvestment in Training**: Comprehensive training programs can be expensive, and facilities under financial pressure may opt for minimal training to cut costs.
- **Cutting Corners on Care**: This might involve rationing supplies, skimping on food quality, or delaying necessary facility maintenance or upgrades.
- **Pressure on Staff**: Staff may face pressure to work faster or take on more responsibilities without additional compensation, potentially leading to rushed or inadequate care.

Case Study: The Orpea Scandal

The investigation into the Orpea Group, one of Europe's largest eldercare providers, revealed how the pursuit of profit could compromise care quality. The company was found to be rationing essential care items, including food and hygiene products, to cut costs and increase profits. This systematic prioritization of financial gain over resident well-being led to widespread neglect and substandard care across numerous facilities.

Public Funding Challenges

While for-profit facilities face unique pressures, publicly funded homes are not immune to financial challenges:

1. **Budget Constraints**: Government-funded facilities often operate under tight budgets, which can limit their ability to invest in staff, training, and resources.
2. **Increasing Costs**: The rising costs of healthcare, coupled with the increasing

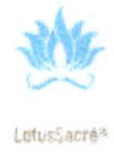

complexity of care needs as people live longer, put strain on fixed budgets.

3. **Political Pressures**: Funding for eldercare can be subject to political whims, leading to uncertainty and potential underfunding.

These challenges can lead to similar issues as seen in for-profit homes, including understaffing, inadequate training, and suboptimal care environments.

Management and Supervision Issues

Even with adequate staffing, training, and funding, poor management and supervision can create an environment where abuse can occur and persist. Key issues include:

Lack of Oversight

1. **Inadequate Monitoring**: Without proper supervision, abusive behaviors may go unnoticed or unchecked.

2. **Failure to Address Complaints**: Management that doesn't take resident or family complaints seriously may allow abusive situations to continue.

3. **Lack of Accountability**: Without clear accountability structures, staff may not feel compelled to maintain high standards of care.

Poor Organizational Culture

1. **Normalization of Substandard Care**: In poorly managed facilities, substandard care practices can become normalized over time.
2. **Lack of Empowerment**: Staff who don't feel empowered to report issues or suggest improvements may become complacent or disengaged.
3. **Prioritizing Procedures Over People**: Management that focuses more on following procedures than on resident well-being can inadvertently create an environment where abuse is more likely.

Ineffective Leadership

1. **Lack of Vision**: Without a clear vision for quality care, facilities may drift towards mediocrity or worse.

2. **Poor Communication**: Ineffective communication between management, staff, residents, and families can lead to misunderstandings and unaddressed issues.
3. **Failure to Lead by Example**: When leadership doesn't model respectful, person-centered care, staff are less likely to prioritize these values.

The impacts of these management and supervision issues can be severe:

- **Persistence of Abuse**: Poor oversight can allow abusive behaviors to continue unchecked.
- **Low Staff Morale**: Poor management often leads to low staff morale, which can result in reduced quality of care and increased risk of abusive behaviors.
- **High Turnover**: Ineffective management often leads to high staff turnover, exacerbating staffing shortages and training issues.
- **Resistance to Change**: Poor organizational culture can make it

LotusSacré

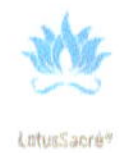

difficult to implement necessary changes or improvements in care practices.

Case Study: The Whistle-blower's Struggle

In a large retirement home in Sydney, Australia, a nurse repeatedly raised concerns about rough handling of residents and medication errors to her supervisors. Her complaints were consistently downplayed or ignored. The lack of response from management not only allowed the abuse to continue but also created a culture where staff felt reporting issues was pointless. This led to widespread underreporting of incidents and a pervasive acceptance of substandard care practices.

The factors contributing to elder abuse in retirement homes - understaffing and insufficient training, financial pressures, and management and supervision issues - are complex and often interrelated. Addressing these systemic issues requires a multifaceted approach involving policy changes, increased funding, improved

LotusSacré

training programs, and a shift in how society values and prioritizes elder care.

It's crucial to recognize that while these factors can create an environment where abuse is more likely to occur, they do not excuse or justify abusive behavior. Individual accountability must go hand in hand with systemic change.

As we move forward, addressing these contributing factors must be a priority in our efforts to combat elder abuse. By tackling these underlying issues, we can create environments where high-quality, respectful care is the norm, and where the dignity and well-being of our elderly population are truly prioritized.

CALL TO ACTION

- Advocate for better working conditions and training for retirement home staff by writing to facility managers and local policymakers.
- Consider supporting or starting a petition for improved staffing ratios in care facilities.

- Organize a community forum to discuss the root causes of elder abuse and brainstorm local solutions.

Please Share Your Thoughts on Amazon!

Your Review Helps:

- Raise awareness about elder abuse in retirement homes
- Support independent authors tackling crucial social issues
- Encourage more research and action on elder care reform

How to Leave a Review:

- Go to the book's Amazon page
- Click "Write a customer review"
- Share your honest thoughts and experiences
- Click submit

If you found value in this book, please consider leaving a 5-star review!

Your support helps fuel further investigation into elder care issues and promotes positive change in our retirement

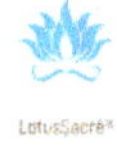

homes. By sharing your thoughts, you're giving a voice to those who often go unheard and contributing to a movement for dignity and respect for our elders.

Together, we can make a difference in the lives of our seniors.

This version maintains the structure and purpose of the original text while adapting the content to fit the theme of your book on elder abuse in retirement homes. It emphasizes the importance of raising awareness about elder abuse and encourages readers to contribute to positive change through their reviews.

CHAPTER 5

CONSEQUENCES OF ABUSE

Elder abuse in retirement homes and long-term care facilities has far-reaching consequences that extend beyond the immediate victims. This chapter explores the multifaceted impact of abuse on the physical and mental health of residents, the profound effects on their families, and the often-overlooked toll on healthcare staff. Understanding these consequences is crucial for comprehending the full scope of this societal issue and developing effective interventions.

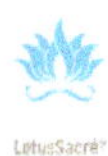
LotusSacré

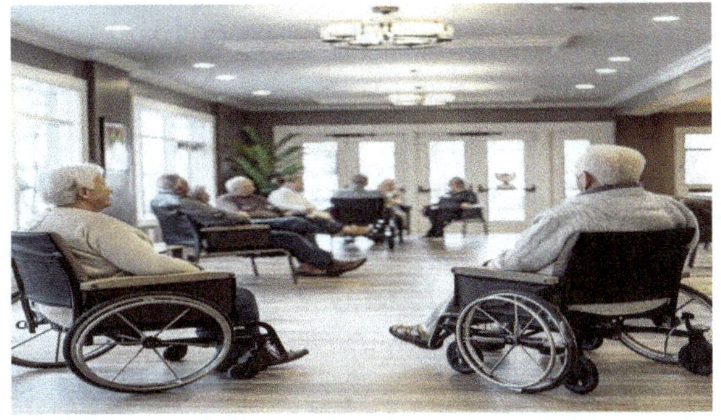

Impact on the Physical and Mental Health of Residents

The effects of abuse on elderly residents are often severe and long-lasting, compromising both their physical and mental well-being.

Physical Health Consequences

1. **Injuries and Physical Trauma**: Physical abuse can result in a range of injuries, from bruises and lacerations to more severe trauma like fractures or internal injuries. These injuries are particularly dangerous for older adults, who may have pre-existing health conditions or reduced ability to heal.

2. **Deterioration of Existing Health Conditions**: Abuse and neglect can exacerbate existing health problems. For instance, failure to provide proper medication or care can lead to the worsening of chronic conditions such as diabetes, heart disease, or arthritis.

3. **Malnutrition and Dehydration**: Neglect often manifests in inadequate nutrition and hydration, leading to weight loss, weakness, and increased susceptibility to illness and infection.

4. **Increased Risk of Mortality**: Studies have shown that elder abuse victims have a significantly higher mortality rate compared to their non-abused peers. The stress and physical toll of abuse can shorten life expectancy.

5. **Decline in Functional Abilities**: Abuse can accelerate the loss of independence in daily activities, leading to increased frailty and dependency.

Mental Health Consequences

1. **Depression and Anxiety**: Abuse often leads to the development or

LotusSacré®

worsening of mental health issues. Feelings of helplessness, fear, and sadness are common, potentially evolving into clinical depression or anxiety disorders.

2. **Post-Traumatic Stress Disorder (PTSD)**: Victims of severe or prolonged abuse may develop PTSD, experiencing flashbacks, nightmares, and severe anxiety related to their traumatic experiences.

3. **Cognitive Decline**: The stress and trauma associated with abuse can accelerate cognitive decline, potentially increasing the risk or progression of dementia.

4. **Low Self-Esteem and Self-Worth**: Constant emotional abuse or neglect can erode an individual's sense of self-worth, leading to feelings of worthlessness and shame.

5. **Social Withdrawal**: Abused residents may become increasingly isolated, withdrawing from social interactions due to fear, shame, or loss of trust in others.

6. **Sleep Disturbances**: Anxiety and fear resulting from abuse can lead to insomnia or other sleep disorders, further impacting overall health and well-being.

7. **Substance Abuse**: In some cases, victims may turn to alcohol or medication abuse as a coping mechanism, further compromising their health.

Consequences for Families

The impact of elder abuse extends beyond the immediate victim, profoundly affecting their family members and loved ones.

Emotional and Psychological Impact

1. **Guilt and Self-Blame**: Family members often experience intense guilt for not preventing the abuse or for placing their loved one in a facility where abuse occurred.

2. **Anger and Frustration**: Discovering that a loved one has been abused can trigger intense anger towards the

perpetrators and the system that allowed it to happen.

3. **Anxiety and Depression**: The emotional toll of dealing with abuse can lead to anxiety and depression among family members, especially if they feel helpless to change the situation.

4. **Trust Issues**: Families may develop a lasting distrust of healthcare institutions and professionals, making future care decisions more challenging.

Family Dynamics and Relationships

1. **Strained Family Relationships**: Disagreements about how to handle the situation can create tension and conflict within families.

2. **Caregiver Burnout**: Family members may take on increased caregiving responsibilities, leading to physical and emotional exhaustion.

3. **Financial Strain**: Legal proceedings, alternative care arrangements, or medical treatments resulting from abuse can place significant financial burdens on families.

Long-Term Effects

1. **Intergenerational Trauma**: The experience of elder abuse can affect how younger family members view aging and care for the elderly, potentially influencing their future decisions and attitudes.
2. **Advocacy and Activism**: Some family members may channel their experiences into becoming advocates for elder rights and improved care standards.
3. **Changes in Family Planning**: The experience may influence how families plan for their own aging or care for other elderly relatives.

Impact on Healthcare Staff

The consequences of elder abuse are not limited to residents and their families; healthcare staff in these facilities are also significantly affected.

Emotional and Psychological Impact

1. **Moral Distress**: Staff who witness abuse but feel powerless to prevent it

often experience significant moral distress, leading to burnout and compassion fatigue.

2. **Secondary Traumatic Stress**: Caregivers who work closely with abuse victims may experience secondary traumatic stress, similar to PTSD, from repeated exposure to others' trauma.

3. **Guilt and Shame**: Staff members who failed to recognize or report abuse may struggle with intense feelings of guilt and shame.

4. **Decreased Job Satisfaction**: The presence of abuse in a facility can significantly reduce job satisfaction and morale among staff.

Professional Consequences

1. **Increased Turnover**: The stress and emotional toll of working in an environment where abuse occurs can lead to higher staff turnover rates.

2. **Legal and Ethical Dilemmas**: Staff may face difficult decisions about reporting abuse, especially if they fear retaliation or job loss.

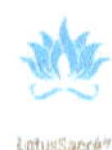

3. **Stigma**: Healthcare workers associated with facilities where abuse has occurred may face stigma in their professional and personal lives.

Impact on Care Quality

1. **Deterioration of Care Standards**: A culture of abuse can lead to a general decline in care standards as staff become desensitized or demoralized.
2. **Communication Breakdown**: Fear and distrust resulting from abuse can hinder effective communication between staff, residents, and families.
3. **Reduced Empathy**: Chronic stress and burnout can lead to reduced empathy among healthcare workers, potentially compromising the quality of care.

Societal Impact

The consequences of elder abuse in care facilities extend beyond individuals and families, affecting society as a whole.

1. **Increased Healthcare Costs**: The physical and mental health consequences of abuse often result in increased healthcare utilization and costs.
2. **Strain on Social Services**: Addressing elder abuse cases puts additional pressure on already strained social services and adult protective services.
3. **Erosion of Trust in Care Systems**: Widespread abuse scandals can erode public trust in the entire elderly care system, making it more challenging to provide necessary care for the aging population.
4. **Legal and Regulatory Challenges**: Abuse cases often lead to legal proceedings and calls for stricter regulations, requiring significant resources and potentially affecting the entire care sector.

The consequences of elder abuse in retirement homes and care facilities are far-reaching and deeply impactful. From the devastating effects on the physical and

mental health of residents to the lasting trauma experienced by families and the professional and personal toll on healthcare staff, the ripple effects of abuse touch every aspect of the care ecosystem. Recognizing these multifaceted consequences is crucial for developing comprehensive strategies to prevent abuse, support victims and their families, and create a culture of compassionate, high-quality care for our elderly population. It underscores the urgent need for systemic changes, improved oversight, and a societal commitment to valuing and protecting our most vulnerable seniors.

CALL TO ACTION

- Share stories of abuse survivors (with their permission) to highlight the real impact of elder abuse.
- Organize a community event to discuss the effects of elder abuse on families and caregivers.
- Create a support group for families affected by elder abuse in care facilities.

Please Share Your Thoughts on Amazon!

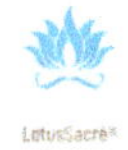

Your Review Helps:

- Raise awareness about elder abuse in retirement homes
- Support independent authors tackling crucial social issues
- Encourage more research and action on elder care reform

How to Leave a Review:

- Go to the book's Amazon page
- Click "Write a customer review"
- Share your honest thoughts and experiences
- Click submit

If you found value in this book, please consider leaving a 5-star review!

Your support helps fuel further investigation into elder care issues and promotes positive change in our retirement homes. By sharing your thoughts, you're giving a voice to those who often go unheard and contributing to a movement for dignity and respect for our elders.

Together, we can make a difference in the lives of our seniors.

This version maintains the structure and purpose of the original text while adapting the content to fit the theme of your book on elder abuse in retirement homes. It emphasizes the importance of raising awareness about elder abuse and encourages readers to contribute to positive change through their reviews.

Please Share Your Thoughts on Amazon!

Your Review Helps:

- Raise awareness about elder abuse in retirement homes
- Support independent authors tackling crucial social issues
- Encourage more research and action on elder care reform

How to Leave a Review:

- Go to the book's Amazon page
- Click "Write a customer review"
- Share your honest thoughts and experiences
- Click submit

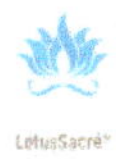

If you found value in this book, please consider leaving a 5-star review!

Your support helps fuel further investigation into elder care issues and promotes positive change in our retirement homes. By sharing your thoughts, you're giving a voice to those who often go unheard and contributing to a movement for dignity and respect for our elders.

Together, we can make a difference in the lives of our seniors.

This version maintains the structure and purpose of the original text while adapting the content to fit the theme of your book on elder abuse in retirement homes. It emphasizes the importance of raising awareness about elder abuse and encourages readers to contribute to positive change through their reviews.

LotusSacré

CHAPTER 6

INTERNATIONAL PERSPECTIVE

Elder abuse in care facilities is a global issue that transcends national borders, cultural differences, and economic divides. This chapter provides a comprehensive exploration of the international landscape of elder care and abuse, offering insights into how different countries approach this complex challenge. By examining diverse systems, analyzing detailed case studies, and highlighting innovative reform initiatives worldwide, we can gain valuable lessons to inform more effective strategies for preventing and addressing elder abuse on a global scale.

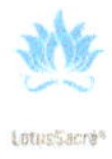

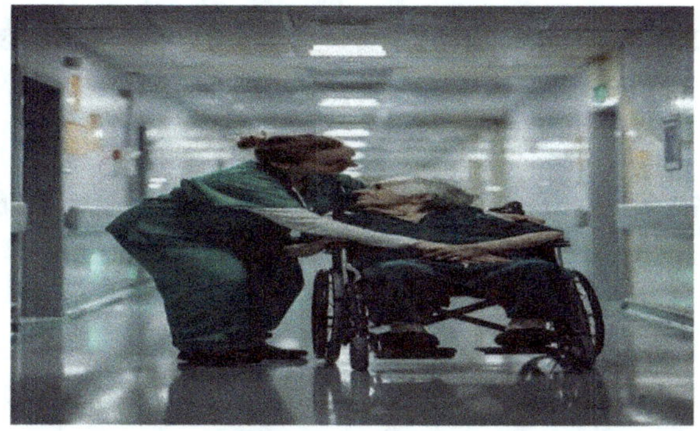

Comparative Analysis of Elder Care Systems and Abuse Prevalence

The prevalence and nature of elder abuse in care facilities vary significantly across countries, influenced by cultural norms, economic factors, healthcare systems, and societal attitudes towards aging. This section provides an in-depth look at several key countries, examining their approaches to elder care and the challenges they face in combating abuse.

United States

The United States faces significant challenges in elder care, with a fragmented system that varies considerably by state. According to the National Council on

Aging, approximately 1 in 10 Americans aged 60+ have experienced some form of elder abuse, with some studies suggesting that the rate in nursing homes and long-term care facilities may be much higher.

Key features of the U.S. system:

- A mix of private and public facilities, with Medicare and Medicaid playing crucial roles in funding
- Mandatory reporting laws for suspected abuse in most states
- Federal oversight through the Centers for Medicare & Medicaid Services (CMS)
- The Elder Justice Act, passed in 2010, which aims to prevent and address elder abuse, neglect, and exploitation

Despite these measures, underreporting remains a significant issue. The National Center on Elder Abuse estimates that only 1 in 14 cases of abuse are reported to authorities. This underreporting is attributed to various factors, including fear of retaliation, lack of awareness, and cognitive impairments among residents.

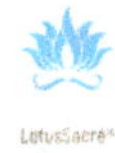

A 2019 study published in the Journal of Elder Abuse & Neglect found that 64% of staff in long-term care facilities admitted to committing some form of abuse in the past year. This startling statistic highlights the pervasive nature of the problem and the urgent need for systemic reforms.

United Kingdom

The UK has been grappling with elder abuse in care homes, particularly in light of high-profile scandals in recent years. The Care Quality Commission (CQC) regulates care homes in England, with similar bodies in Scotland (Care Inspectorate), Wales (Care Inspectorate Wales), and Northern Ireland (Regulation and Quality Improvement Authority).

Key aspects of the UK system:

- A national health service (NHS) that provides some long-term care, supplemented by private facilities
- Mandatory safeguarding procedures for vulnerable adults

- Regular inspections by regulatory bodies like the CQC
- The Care Act 2014, which places adult safeguarding on a statutory footing

A report by Age UK suggests that up to 500,000 older people in the UK may be subject to abuse or neglect each year, with a significant portion occurring in care settings. The CQC's 2019/2020 report revealed that 1% of care homes were rated as "inadequate" and 15% as "requires improvement" in terms of safety, indicating ongoing challenges in ensuring quality care.

The UK has also been at the forefront of addressing financial abuse in care settings. The Office of the Public Guardian, established under the Mental Capacity Act 2005, plays a crucial role in protecting vulnerable adults from financial exploitation.

Germany

Germany's approach to elder care is often cited as a model for other countries. The

country introduced long-term care insurance in 1995, which has helped to fund a comprehensive system of care.

Notable features of the German system:

- Mandatory long-term care insurance for all citizens
- A strong emphasis on home care and community-based services
- Stringent regulations and regular inspections of care facilities
- The Pflegestärkungsgesetze (Care Strengthening Acts), a series of reforms implemented between 2015 and 2017 to improve care quality

Despite these measures, studies suggest that elder abuse remains a concern in Germany. A 2018 study by the German Center of Gerontology estimated that between 5% to 10% of older adults in Germany experience some form of mistreatment, including those in care facilities.

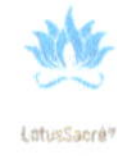

Germany's approach to workforce development in elder care is particularly noteworthy. The country has implemented comprehensive training programs for care workers, including a three-year vocational training course for elder care professionals. This focus on professionalization aims to improve care quality and reduce the risk of abuse through better-trained staff.

Japan

As the country with the world's oldest population, Japan's approach to elder care is of particular interest. The country introduced a comprehensive long-term care insurance system in 2000, which has since undergone several revisions to address changing demographics and care needs.

Key elements of Japan's system:

- Universal long-term care insurance
- A cultural emphasis on filial piety, which can sometimes mask abuse
- Innovative use of technology in care settings to prevent and detect abuse

- The "Community-based Integrated Care System," which aims to provide seamless health care and long-term care in communities

While official statistics on elder abuse in Japanese care facilities are limited, a 2020 government survey found that about 17,000 cases of abuse by caregivers were reported in a single year, with experts believing this to be an underestimate. The Japanese government has responded with initiatives such as the Elder Abuse Prevention Law, enacted in 2006, which mandates the reporting of suspected abuse cases.

Japan's approach to addressing the challenges of an aging population extends beyond traditional care models. The country has been a pioneer in developing care robots and other assistive technologies to supplement human caregivers, potentially reducing the risk of abuse stemming from caregiver stress and burnout.

Case Studies: Universal Challenges and Unique Regional Issues

Examining specific cases from around the world can provide valuable insights into both common challenges and unique regional issues in addressing elder abuse in care facilities. These case studies offer a more nuanced understanding of the complexities involved in preventing and addressing elder abuse across different cultural and societal contexts.

Case Study 1: Staffing Shortages in Swedish Nursing Homes

In 2020, Sweden faced international criticism for its handling of COVID-19 in nursing homes, which highlighted long-standing issues of understaffing and inadequate training. This case underscores how systemic problems can lead to neglect and substandard care, even in countries known for strong social welfare systems.

Background: Sweden has long been regarded as a model welfare state, with a

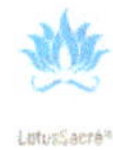

comprehensive system of elder care. However, the COVID-19 pandemic exposed significant weaknesses in the system, particularly in nursing homes.

Key issues:

- Chronic understaffing in many facilities
- High proportion of part-time and temporary workers
- Inadequate training, especially in infection control measures
- Lack of personal protective equipment (PPE) during the pandemic

Consequences:

- High mortality rates among nursing home residents during the pandemic
- Increased instances of neglect due to staff overwhelm
- Public outcry and calls for systemic reform

Key learnings:

- The critical importance of adequate staffing ratios

LotusSacré

- The need for ongoing training and support for care workers
- The potential consequences of prioritizing efficiency over quality of care
- The importance of robust emergency preparedness plans in care facilities

This case highlights how even well-regarded systems can have underlying issues that, when exposed by a crisis, can lead to severe consequences for vulnerable older adults.

Case Study 2: Financial Abuse in Australian Aged Care Facilities

A royal commission into aged care quality and safety in Australia, conducted from 2018 to 2021, uncovered widespread financial abuse in care homes, including overcharging and misuse of residents' funds. This case highlights the complex nature of elder abuse, extending beyond physical and emotional mistreatment.

Background: Australia's aged care system has been under scrutiny for years, with concerns about quality of care and financial management. The royal commission was established in response to a series of scandals and public concerns.

Key findings:

- Instances of facilities charging for services not provided
- Misuse of residents' personal funds by staff members
- Complex fee structures that confused residents and families
- Inadequate financial oversight and auditing processes

Consequences:

- Financial losses for many elderly residents
- Erosion of trust in the aged care system
- Calls for major reforms in the sector

Key insights:

- The need for robust financial oversight in care facilities
- The importance of educating residents and families about financial rights
- The role of regulatory bodies in preventing financial exploitation
- The potential for technology to improve transparency in financial management

This case study demonstrates that elder abuse is not limited to physical or emotional mistreatment, and that financial abuse can have severe impacts on the well-being and dignity of older adults in care.

Case Study 3: Cultural Factors in Elder Abuse in India

In India, where traditional family-based care is giving way to institutional care in urban areas, a study in Delhi nursing homes revealed how cultural factors can influence the manifestation and reporting of elder abuse. Issues such as stigma around institutional care and cultural

norms of respect for elders complicated the identification and addressing of abuse.

Background: India is experiencing rapid population aging alongside urbanization and changing family structures. This has led to an increase in institutional care, a concept that conflicts with traditional values of filial piety.

Key issues:

- Stigma associated with placing elders in care homes
- Cultural reluctance to discuss or report abuse
- Lack of culturally appropriate assessment tools for abuse
- Limited regulatory oversight of care facilities

Findings:

- Underreporting of abuse due to shame and fear of family dishonor
- Forms of abuse influenced by cultural norms (e.g., withholding traditional foods as punishment)

- Staff often untrained in recognizing culturally-specific forms of abuse
- Residents reluctant to complain due to cultural emphasis on respecting authority

Lessons learned:

- The need for culturally sensitive approaches to detecting and preventing abuse
- The importance of community engagement in oversight of care facilities
- The role of public education in changing attitudes towards elder care and abuse
- The necessity of developing culturally appropriate assessment tools and intervention strategies

This case study underscores the importance of considering cultural contexts when addressing elder abuse, particularly in societies undergoing rapid social change.

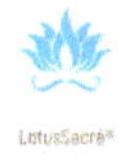

Innovative International Initiatives and Reforms

Countries around the world are implementing innovative approaches to combat elder abuse in care facilities. These initiatives demonstrate the potential for creative solutions to address this complex issue.

1. Technology-Driven Monitoring in the Netherlands

The Netherlands has pioneered the use of smart technology in care homes. Some facilities use sensor systems to monitor residents' movements and alert staff to potential falls or unusual patterns that might indicate abuse or neglect.

Specific initiatives:

- The "Smart Floor" system, which uses pressure-sensitive tiles to detect falls and movement patterns
- Acoustic monitoring systems that can detect sounds of distress

- AI-powered video analysis to identify potential abuse situations while maintaining privacy

Impact:

- Reduced response times to emergencies
- Improved detection of patterns that might indicate abuse
- Enhanced sense of security for residents and families
- Potential for early intervention in abuse situations

Challenges:

- Balancing surveillance with privacy concerns
- Ensuring staff are properly trained to use and interpret data from these systems
- High initial costs of implementation

The Dutch approach demonstrates how technology can be leveraged to create safer care environments while respecting residents' dignity and privacy.

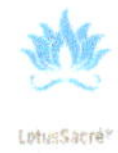

2. Intergenerational Care Programs in Singapore

Singapore has introduced programs that combine preschools with nursing homes, fostering intergenerational interaction. This approach has shown promise in improving the quality of life for older adults and creating a more open, community-oriented care environment less prone to abuse.

Key features:

- Co-located facilities for children and older adults
- Structured intergenerational activities and shared spaces
- Training for staff in both elder care and early childhood education
- Community involvement in facility activities

Benefits:

- Increased social engagement for older adults
- Greater community oversight of care facilities

- Improved empathy and understanding between generations
- Enhanced cognitive stimulation for older adults
- Reduced isolation and depression among residents

Challenges:

- Ensuring appropriate boundaries and safety measures
- Managing diverse needs of different age groups
- Overcoming initial skepticism from families and community members

Singapore's intergenerational care model offers a unique approach to creating more vibrant, connected care environments that may naturally deter abuse through increased transparency and community involvement.

3. Rights-Based Approach in Canada

Canada has implemented a rights-based approach to elder care in some provinces, emphasizing resident autonomy and

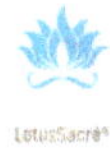
LotusSacré

dignity. This includes initiatives like resident councils in care homes and mandatory rights education for staff and residents.

Key elements:

- Residents' Bill of Rights enshrined in provincial legislation
- Mandatory residents' councils in long-term care homes
- Regular rights education sessions for staff, residents, and families
- Ombudsman programs specifically for long-term care residents

Outcomes:

- Empowerment of residents to advocate for themselves
- Increased awareness of rights among staff and families
- Reduction in reported cases of abuse and neglect
- Improved communication between residents, families, and staff

Challenges:

- Ensuring meaningful participation of residents with cognitive impairments
- Overcoming institutional resistance to increased resident autonomy
- Balancing individual rights with health and safety concerns

Canada's rights-based approach demonstrates how empowering residents and raising awareness of rights can create a culture of respect and dignity in care settings.

4. Comprehensive Staff Support in Denmark

Denmark has focused on improving working conditions and support for care staff as a means of preventing abuse. This includes higher pay, better staff-to-resident ratios, and comprehensive mental health support for caregivers.

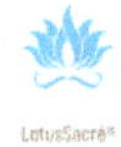

Key initiatives:

- Competitive salaries and benefits for care workers
- Mandatory staff-to-resident ratios
- Regular supervision and mental health check-ins for staff
- Comprehensive training programs, including stress management and conflict resolution

Results:

- Lower staff turnover rates
- Improved quality of care
- Reduced incidence of burnout-related neglect and abuse
- Increased job satisfaction among care workers

Challenges:

- Higher costs of care provision
- Ensuring consistent implementation across different facilities
- Addressing societal attitudes towards care work

Denmark's approach highlights the importance of addressing the root causes of abuse, including staff stress and burnout, through comprehensive support systems.

The global perspective on elder abuse in care facilities reveals both the universality of certain challenges and the diversity of approaches in addressing them. While the prevalence of abuse remains a serious concern worldwide, innovative initiatives and reforms offer hope for improvement.

Key takeaways from this international overview include:

1. The importance of robust regulatory frameworks and oversight
2. The potential of technology in monitoring and preventing abuse
3. The value of community engagement and intergenerational programs
4. The critical role of staff support and training in preventing abuse
5. The need for culturally sensitive approaches to care and abuse prevention

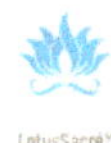

6. The effectiveness of rights-based approaches in empowering residents
7. The potential for financial oversight to prevent economic exploitation
8. The importance of addressing systemic issues like staffing shortages

By learning from international experiences and best practices, countries can work towards creating care systems that not only prevent abuse but also enhance the dignity, autonomy, and quality of life of older adults in care facilities. The global nature of this challenge calls for continued international collaboration and knowledge sharing to protect our most vulnerable elderly populations.

As societies worldwide continue to age, the imperative to address elder abuse in care settings becomes ever more pressing. The diverse approaches highlighted in this chapter demonstrate that there is no one-size-fits-all solution. Instead, effective strategies must be tailored to local contexts while drawing on global best practices. By combining technological innovations,

cultural sensitivity, rights-based approaches, and comprehensive staff support, we can work towards a future where elder abuse in care facilities becomes increasingly rare, and where older adults can age with dignity, respect, and security.

CALL TO ACTION

- Research elder care policies in other countries and share best practices with local policymakers.
- Join international elder rights forums to connect with advocates worldwide.
- Organize a webinar or local event featuring speakers from different countries to discuss global elder care practices.

Please Share Your Thoughts on Amazon!

Your Review Helps:

- Raise awareness about elder abuse in retirement homes
- Support independent authors tackling crucial social issues
- Encourage more research and action on elder care reform

How to Leave a Review:

- Go to the book's Amazon page
- Click "Write a customer review"
- Share your honest thoughts and experiences
- Click submit

If you found value in this book, please consider leaving a 5-star review!

Your support helps fuel further investigation into elder care issues and promotes positive change in our retirement homes. By sharing your thoughts, you're giving a voice to those who often go unheard and contributing to a movement for dignity and respect for our elders.

Together, we can make a difference in the lives of our seniors.

This version maintains the structure and purpose of the original text while adapting the content to fit the theme of your book on elder abuse in retirement homes. It emphasizes the importance of raising awareness about elder abuse and encourages readers to contribute to positive change through their reviews.

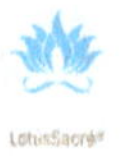

CHAPTER 7:

ANSWERS AND SOLUTIONS

The challenge of elder abuse in care facilities demands a comprehensive and nuanced response that addresses both its immediate manifestations and underlying causes. As we've explored throughout this book, the problem is complex and multifaceted, requiring solutions that are equally sophisticated and far-reaching. This chapter examines the various approaches being implemented around the world to combat elder abuse and improve the quality of life for older adults in care settings, focusing on legislative reforms, community initiatives, and innovative practices that have shown promise in addressing this critical issue.

LotusSacre

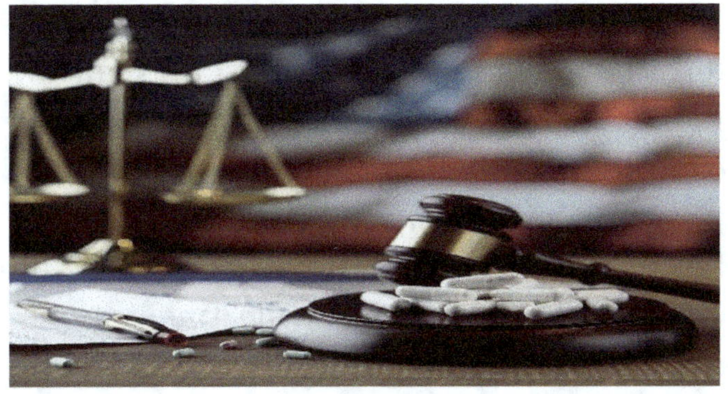

Legislative and Regulatory Reforms

The legal framework surrounding elder care plays a crucial role in preventing and addressing abuse. Over the past several decades, many countries have strengthened their legislative approaches to protecting vulnerable older adults in care facilities. These reforms reflect a growing understanding of the complexities of elder abuse and the need for robust legal protections.

In the United States, the Elder Justice Act of 2010 marked a significant milestone in the federal response to elder abuse. This comprehensive legislation not only mandated reporting of suspected crimes

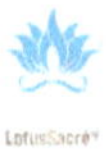

against residents in federally funded long-term care facilities but also established the Elder Justice Coordinating Council to coordinate activities related to elder abuse across federal agencies. The Act provides funding for adult protective services and creates a framework for collecting national data on elder abuse, neglect, and exploitation. While implementation has faced challenges, particularly regarding funding, the Act represents a crucial step toward addressing elder abuse at a systemic level.

Australia's approach to legislative reform has been similarly comprehensive. The 2007 amendment to the Aged Care Act made reporting of serious incidents in residential care mandatory, but perhaps more significantly, it established the Aged Care Quality and Safety Commission as an independent regulator. This body has broad powers to conduct unannounced inspections, investigate complaints, and enforce compliance with quality standards. The effectiveness of this regulatory approach was tested during the COVID-19

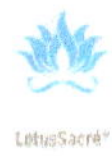

pandemic, leading to further reforms that strengthened the Commission's powers and increased transparency in the aged care sector.

Enhanced oversight through regular inspections has proven to be a critical component of effective regulatory frameworks. England's Care Quality Commission (CQC) has developed a sophisticated approach to monitoring care facilities that goes beyond simple compliance checks. The CQC's inspection regime evaluates services across five key questions: are they safe, effective, caring, responsive, and well-led? This holistic approach recognizes that abuse is often symptomatic of broader organizational failings. The Commission's public reporting system not only helps identify issues but also empowers families to make informed decisions about care options and creates market pressures for improvement.

The qualification and training of care staff has emerged as another crucial area for legislative attention. Germany's approach

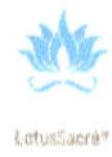

to professional standards in elder care offers valuable insights. The country's Care Qualification Ordinance establishes a comprehensive framework for training care workers, requiring a three-year vocational program that combines theoretical education with practical experience. This emphasis on professionalization not only improves the quality of care but also helps to prevent abuse by ensuring that staff are properly equipped to handle the challenges of elder care. Similarly, Japan's Certified Care Worker qualification, which requires extensive education and successful completion of a national examination, reflects an understanding that high-quality care requires skilled and knowledgeable practitioners.

Many jurisdictions have also recognized the importance of explicitly establishing and protecting the rights of care facility residents. Ontario, Canada's Long-Term Care Homes Act includes a comprehensive Residents' Bill of Rights that goes beyond basic protections against abuse and neglect. It affirms residents' rights to privacy,

dignity, autonomy, and participation in decisions affecting their care. The Act requires care homes to prominently display these rights and provide regular education sessions for staff, residents, and families. This rights-based approach helps to create a culture of respect and empowerment that can serve as a bulwark against abusive practices.

NGO Initiatives and Community Engagement

While legislative reforms provide an essential framework for addressing elder abuse, the role of non-governmental organizations and community initiatives cannot be overstated. These grassroots efforts often provide the practical implementation and human connection that bring policies to life and create real change on the ground.

The International Network for the Prevention of Elder Abuse (INPEA) has been at the forefront of global efforts to raise awareness about elder abuse. Through

its annual World Elder Abuse Awareness Day, observed on June 15th, INPEA has helped to create a global conversation about elder abuse and promoted the exchange of knowledge and best practices across borders. The organization's work illustrates the importance of awareness-raising in combating a problem that often thrives in silence and shadows.

Direct support services provided by NGOs form another crucial line of defense against elder abuse. In the United Kingdom, The Silver Line offers a free, confidential helpline for older adults that operates 24 hours a day, 365 days a year. While not exclusively focused on abuse, the helpline provides a vital point of contact for isolated older adults and can serve as an early warning system for identifying potential abuse. The organization also offers befriending services that help to combat the social isolation that can make older adults more vulnerable to abuse.

Community engagement initiatives have shown particular promise in prevention

and early intervention. Intergenerational programs, pioneered in countries like Singapore and the Netherlands, challenge the segregation of older adults that can contribute to their vulnerability to abuse. These programs, which bring together care home residents with young children for regular activities, create more open and transparent care environments. The presence of children, their families, and teachers in care facilities increases community oversight and creates connections that can make abuse less likely to occur and more likely to be detected if it does.

Innovative Practices and Technological Solutions

The field of elder care has seen significant innovations in recent years, particularly in the application of technology to prevent and detect abuse. The Netherlands has been at the forefront of these developments, pioneering the use of smart monitoring systems in care homes. These systems use a combination of sensors,

artificial intelligence, and human oversight to detect unusual patterns that might indicate abuse or neglect. For example, some facilities employ acoustic monitoring systems that can identify sounds of distress while respecting privacy, or movement sensors that can detect if a resident has fallen or is experiencing unusual patterns of activity.

While the implementation of such technology must be carefully balanced with privacy concerns and the dignity of residents, early results suggest that these systems can contribute to safer care environments. The key lies in using technology to support and enhance human care, rather than replace it. When properly implemented, these systems can help to alleviate the burden on staff and allow them to focus more on providing high-quality, person-centered care.

Beyond technological solutions, innovative staffing and support models have shown promise in reducing the incidence of abuse. Denmark's comprehensive approach to

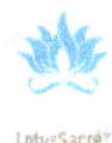

staff support, for instance, recognizes that preventing abuse requires addressing the conditions that can lead caregivers to engage in abusive behavior. The Danish model includes competitive salaries, manageable workloads, and regular supervision and mental health support for caregivers. By addressing issues like burnout and job dissatisfaction, this approach has led to lower staff turnover rates and improved quality of care.

Rights-based approaches to care, as implemented in some Canadian provinces, represent another innovative practice. These approaches go beyond simply protecting residents from abuse to actively promoting their autonomy and dignity. Regular rights education sessions for staff, residents, and families create a culture of respect and empowerment. The establishment of resident councils gives older adults a voice in the operation of their care facilities and creates channels for addressing concerns before they escalate to abuse.

Measuring Success and Adapting Solutions

As we consider the various approaches to addressing elder abuse, it's crucial to acknowledge the challenges of measuring their effectiveness. The hidden nature of much elder abuse, combined with underreporting and the difficulty of conducting research in care settings, can make it hard to definitively evaluate the impact of different interventions.

However, some promising indicators have emerged. In jurisdictions with strong regulatory frameworks and regular inspections, there is evidence of improved compliance with care standards and quicker identification of potential issues. Community engagement initiatives have been associated with increased reporting of concerns and greater family involvement in care. Staff support programs have led to measurable improvements in job satisfaction and retention, factors that are likely to contribute to better care and reduced risk of abuse.

The key to successful intervention appears to lie in the combination of multiple approaches. Strong legislation provides the necessary framework, but it must be accompanied by robust enforcement and practical support for implementation. Community engagement creates transparency and connection, while technological innovations can provide additional safeguards. Underlying all of these approaches must be a commitment to person-centered care that respects the dignity and autonomy of older adults.

The Way Forward

As we look to the future, several key principles emerge for advancing the fight against elder abuse in care facilities:

1. **Comprehensive Approaches:** Effective solutions must address multiple aspects of the problem, from legal protections to staff support to community engagement.
2. **Person-Centered Care:** All interventions should be grounded in

respect for the dignity and autonomy of older adults.

3. **Evidence-Based Practice:** Continued research and evaluation are essential for identifying the most effective approaches and adapting them to different contexts.

4. **Cultural Sensitivity:** Solutions must be adaptable to different cultural contexts while maintaining core principles of respect and protection.

5. **Preventive Focus:** While responding to abuse remains crucial, preventing it from occurring in the first place should be the ultimate goal.

The path to eliminating elder abuse in care facilities is long and complex, but the range of solutions being implemented around the world offers hope for progress. By combining strong legislation, community involvement, technological innovation, and a commitment to best practices, we can work towards creating care environments where older adults can live with dignity, respect, and security. The challenge ahead lies in scaling up successful interventions,

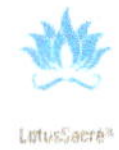

adapting them to different contexts, and maintaining the political and social will to prioritize the protection of vulnerable older adults.

As our societies continue to age, the imperative to address elder abuse grows ever more pressing. The solutions discussed in this chapter demonstrate that while the challenge is significant, it is not insurmountable. Through continued collaboration, innovation, and commitment to the dignity of older adults, we can work towards a future where elder abuse in care facilities becomes increasingly rare, and where the final years of life are characterized by security, respect, and well-being.

CALL TO ACTION

- Get involved with local NGOs working on elder rights.
- Share success stories of reform in elder care to inspire change in your community.

- Develop a "best practices" guide for local care facilities based on successful models from around the world.

Please Share Your Thoughts on Amazon!

Your Review Helps:

- Raise awareness about elder abuse in retirement homes
- Support independent authors tackling crucial social issues
- Encourage more research and action on elder care reform

How to Leave a Review:

- Go to the book's Amazon page
- Click "Write a customer review"
- Share your honest thoughts and experiences
- Click submit

If you found value in this book, please consider leaving a 5-star review!

Your support helps fuel further investigation into elder care issues and promotes positive change in our retirement

homes. By sharing your thoughts, you're giving a voice to those who often go unheard and contributing to a movement for dignity and respect for our elders.

Together, we can make a difference in the lives of our seniors.

This version maintains the structure and purpose of the original text while adapting the content to fit the theme of your book on elder abuse in retirement homes. It emphasizes the importance of raising awareness about elder abuse and encourages readers to contribute to positive change through their reviews.

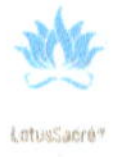

CHAPTER 8

ROLE OF YOUNG ADULTS

In the ongoing battle against elder abuse in retirement homes, an unexpected yet powerful ally has emerged: young adults. While conversations about elder care typically focus on healthcare professionals, policymakers, and family members directly affected by aging relatives, the role of younger generations in preventing and addressing elder abuse has become increasingly significant.

This chapter explores how young adults, typically aged 18-35, are contributing to positive changes in retirement homes through three key avenues: awareness and education, commitment and volunteering, and preparation for their own aging future. Young adults bring unique perspectives and abilities to the challenge of elder abuse prevention. Their technological literacy, energy, and fresh outlook on long-standing issues make them valuable assets in improving retirement home conditions. Moreover, their involvement creates a bridge between generations, fostering understanding and empathy that can help prevent abuse and enhance the quality of life for elderly residents.

As we get into each aspect of young adult involvement, we'll discover how their participation not only benefits current elderly residents but also shapes a future where retirement homes can better serve an aging population. Their role represents more than just an additional resource; it symbolizes a shift in how society approaches elder care and abuse prevention.

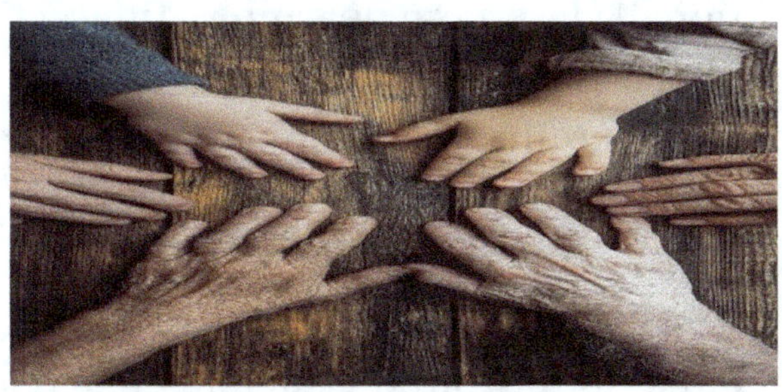

Awareness and Education

The journey toward combating elder abuse in retirement homes begins with awareness and education among young adults. As our society grapples with this growing crisis, engaging younger generations in understanding and recognizing the signs of elder abuse has become crucial. Universities and colleges are increasingly incorporating modules on elder care and abuse prevention into various curricula, not just in healthcare-related fields but also in social work, law, and even business programs.

These educational initiatives go beyond traditional classroom learning. Interactive workshops, seminars, and real-world exposure to retirement home environments help young adults develop a deeper understanding of the challenges faced by elderly residents. For instance, nursing programs now often include extensive training on recognizing subtle signs of abuse or neglect, while law students learn about the legal frameworks protecting

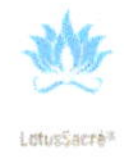

elderly rights and the complexities of elder abuse cases.

Social media has emerged as a powerful tool for raising awareness among young adults. Platforms like Instagram and TikTok, typically associated with youth culture, are now being used to share information about elder abuse prevention. Young influencers collaborate with elder rights organizations to create engaging content that educates their peers about the importance of quality elder care and the warning signs of abuse.

Educational institutions are also partnering with retirement homes to create immersive learning experiences. These partnerships allow students to interact directly with elderly residents and care staff, gaining firsthand insights into the daily realities of retirement home life. Such experiences often prove transformative, changing young adults' perspectives on aging and elder care.

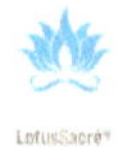

Commitment and Volunteering

The awareness fostered through education naturally leads to increased commitment and volunteering among young adults. Many are now actively seeking opportunities to contribute their time and skills to improving the lives of elderly residents in retirement homes. This commitment manifests in various forms, from regular visitation programs to more structured volunteer initiatives.

Volunteer programs specifically designed for young adults are gaining popularity in retirement homes. These programs go beyond traditional activities like reading to residents or organizing events. Young volunteers are now involved in more sophisticated roles, such as:

- Providing technology assistance to help residents stay connected with family
- Organizing intergenerational activities that benefit both residents and volunteers

- Participating in monitoring programs to ensure quality of care
- Supporting staff in various capacities, bringing fresh energy to the environment

Universities and colleges often facilitate these volunteer opportunities through service-learning programs, allowing students to earn credits while making meaningful contributions to elder care. This academic integration ensures that volunteering is not just an extracurricular activity but a valued part of young adults' educational experience.

The commitment of young volunteers has multiple positive effects on retirement homes. Their presence brings vibrancy and energy to the environment, and their regular involvement creates an additional layer of oversight that can help prevent abuse. Many retirement homes report that the presence of young volunteers improves the overall atmosphere and resident engagement.

Bridging Generations: Young Adults as Champions for Elder Care

In a quaint café in downtown Paris, 23-year-old Marie Dupont sips her coffee while video chatting with her grandmother, who resides in a retirement home two hours away. This weekly ritual, born from a place of love and duty, represents a growing movement among young adults who are actively engaging with elderly care issues. Marie's story, like many others, illustrates a pivotal shift in how younger generations view their role in supporting and protecting older adults.

The relationship between young adults and elder care is undergoing a profound transformation. As our global population ages, the importance of intergenerational connections becomes increasingly apparent. Young adults, often perceived as disconnected from issues affecting the elderly, are emerging as powerful advocates and change-makers in the fight against elder abuse and neglect.

Twenty-six-year-old Thomas Lefebvre never imagined he would become an advocate for elder rights. His journey began when he witnessed concerning conditions during visits to his great-aunt's retirement home. "At first, I felt powerless," Thomas recalls. "But then I realized that my generation's technological savvy and social media presence could be powerful tools for change." Thomas started a blog documenting his observations and connecting with other young adults sharing similar experiences. His platform quickly evolved into a community where younger people could learn about elder care issues and find ways to make a difference.

The digital native generation brings unique perspectives and skills to elder advocacy. Social media campaigns, online petitions, and viral videos have become powerful weapons in exposing elder abuse and rallying support for better care standards. When 28-year-old software developer Sarah Chen created an app allowing families to track and rate the quality of care in retirement homes, she demonstrated

how young innovators could leverage technology to address age-old problems.

Universities across France are taking notice of this emerging trend. The University of Lyon recently introduced a course titled "Intergenerational Studies: Bridging the Age Gap," which has become unexpectedly popular among students from various disciplines. Professor Claire Moreau, who teaches the course, notes, "Young adults today understand that elder care isn't just a family issue or a healthcare issue—it's a societal issue that affects us all."

The volunteering landscape in retirement homes is also evolving. Gone are the days when young volunteers simply served tea or played cards with residents. Today's young adults are initiating art therapy sessions, teaching digital literacy classes, and even conducting oral history projects to preserve residents' stories. These interactions not only enrich the lives of elderly residents but also provide young volunteers with valuable perspectives on aging and life.

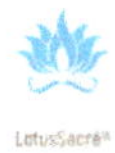

Lucas Martin, a 24-year-old nursing student, splits his time between his studies and volunteering at a local EHPAD (Établissement d'Hébergement pour Personnes Âgées Dépendantes). "Every hour I spend with the residents teaches me something my textbooks can't," he explains. "They've shown me that good elder care isn't just about medical expertise—it's about dignity, respect, and human connection."

Yet, awareness and volunteering are just the beginning. Young adults are increasingly recognizing the importance of preparing for their own aging process and that of their loved ones. Financial advisors report a surge in millennials seeking information about long-term care insurance and retirement planning. This forward-thinking approach stems from witnessing the challenges their grandparents face and a determination to create better outcomes for future generations.

Emma Rousseau, a 29-year-old architect, has already started discussions with her parents about their future care preferences. "It might seem premature," she admits, "but I've seen how lack of planning can lead to hasty decisions in crisis situations. I want to ensure my parents' wishes are known and respected." Emma's proactive approach reflects a growing awareness among young adults that elder care planning should begin long before it becomes an immediate necessity.

The impact of young adult involvement extends beyond individual actions. Youth-led organizations advocating for elder rights have gained significant traction in recent years. The "Grands-Parents & Petits-Enfants Unis" (Grandparents & Grandchildren United) movement, founded by university students, has successfully lobbied for stricter oversight of retirement homes and better training for care staff.

These young advocates have also brought fresh perspectives to the conversation about elder abuse. Rather than viewing it

solely as a problem to be solved, they emphasize the importance of creating positive alternatives. Innovation competitions focused on improving elder care have attracted young entrepreneurs eager to develop solutions. From AI-powered monitoring systems to community engagement platforms, these innovations reflect a generation's commitment to ensuring dignity in aging.

However, the journey is not without its challenges. Young adults often face skepticism from older professionals in the elder care sector. "Sometimes, our age is seen as a limitation rather than an asset," says Philippe Dubois, a 25-year-old geriatric care consultant. "But we're not trying to replace existing expertise—we're trying to complement it with fresh energy and new approaches."

The COVID-19 pandemic highlighted both the vulnerabilities of elderly populations and the potential of young adult advocacy. When retirement homes went into lockdown, young volunteers organized

tablet donation drives to help residents stay connected with their families. Others created online platforms where retirement home staff could share best practices for preventing virus transmission while maintaining quality of care.

As young adults engage more deeply with elder care issues, many find their career aspirations shifting. Medical schools report increased interest in geriatric specializations, while social work programs see more students focusing on elder care policy. This influx of young professionals brings new energy and perspectives to a sector traditionally challenged by staff shortages and burnout.

Education about elder care issues is also evolving to reach younger audiences earlier. Some high schools have introduced community service programs partnering students with local retirement homes. These experiences often spark a lifelong interest in elder advocacy and help dispel stereotypes about aging and elder care.

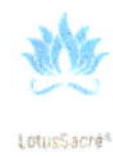

Looking ahead, the role of young adults in addressing elder abuse and improving elder care continues to expand. As Marie Dupont finishes her video call with her grandmother, she reflects on the future. "Our generation has the power to reshape how society views and treats its elderly members," she says. "It's not just about preventing abuse—it's about creating a world where every stage of life is valued and protected."

The involvement of young adults in elder care represents more than just a demographic shift—it's a reimagining of intergenerational relationships and responsibilities. As they bring their energy, technological expertise, and fresh perspectives to the field, young adults are not just preparing for their own futures; they are actively working to create a society where dignity in aging is not just an ideal, but a reality.

Through awareness, education, commitment, and forward planning, young adults are proving that elder care is not just

a concern for the old, but a calling for the young. Their engagement offers hope for a future where retirement homes are not places of potential abuse and neglect, but communities of respect, care, and intergenerational connection.

The Vital Role of Young Adults in Combating Elder Abuse

In the complex landscape of elder care and abuse prevention, an unexpected yet powerful force for change has emerged: young adults. As our society grapples with the growing crisis of elder abuse in retirement homes, the engagement of younger generations has become not just beneficial, but essential. This chapter explores how young adults are becoming pivotal agents of change in the fight against elder abuse, bridging generational gaps and bringing fresh perspectives to an age-old problem.

The relationship between young adults and the elderly has traditionally been viewed through the lens of family bonds —

grandchildren visiting grandparents, sharing holiday meals, or occasionally helping with errands. However, a more profound and systemic connection is developing as young people increasingly recognize the broader societal implications of elder abuse and take active steps to combat it.

Sarah Chen, a 24-year-old nursing student, exemplifies this new wave of engagement. During her clinical rotations, she witnessed firsthand the challenges faced by elderly residents in care facilities. "I saw how a simple conversation could brighten someone's day," she recalls. "But I also noticed the warning signs of neglect that others might miss." Motivated by her experiences, Sarah started a volunteer program at her university, connecting students with local retirement homes. The initiative has grown from five volunteers to over fifty in just two years, creating a network of young advocates for elder care quality.

This growing awareness among young adults isn't happening in isolation. Social media platforms have become powerful tools for education and advocacy. Hashtags like #ElderRights and #AgeismAwareness have gained traction, with young influencers using their platforms to shine a light on issues facing the elderly population. These digital natives are leveraging their technological savvy to amplify voices that have long gone unheard.

The impact of this increased awareness extends beyond social media activism. Young professionals entering fields such as healthcare, law, and social work are bringing with them a heightened sensitivity to elder abuse issues. Law schools report a growing interest in elder law, while medical schools are expanding their geriatric care curricula in response to student demand. This shift suggests that the next generation of professionals will be better equipped to recognize, prevent, and address elder abuse in institutional settings.

The commitment of young adults to this cause often manifests in innovative ways. Take Marcus Thompson, a 28-year-old software developer who created an app that helps families stay connected with their elderly relatives in care homes. The app not only facilitates communication but also includes features for tracking care quality and reporting concerns. "Technology can bridge gaps," Marcus explains. "We can use it to ensure our elders are treated with the dignity they deserve."

Volunteering has become another crucial avenue for young adult involvement. Beyond traditional activities like reading to residents or organizing events, young volunteers are taking on more sophisticated roles. They're conducting social media campaigns, participating in advocacy efforts, and even serving on advisory boards for retirement homes. This level of engagement not only benefits the elderly residents but also provides young adults with valuable experiences and insights.

The presence of young volunteers in retirement homes has multiple positive effects. Staff members report that the energy and enthusiasm of young adults can transform the atmosphere of a facility. Residents often become more engaged and communicative when interacting with younger visitors. Moreover, the regular presence of outside observers can serve as a deterrent to potential abuse, creating an additional layer of informal oversight.

However, the relationship between young adults and elder care isn't just about what young people can give – it's also about what they can learn. Through their involvement with elderly care issues, many young adults report gaining new perspectives on aging, vulnerability, and the importance of dignified care. This understanding is crucial as they begin to think about their own futures and the kind of society they want to grow old in.

Lisa Okonjo, a 31-year-old social worker, reflects on this dual benefit: "Working with elderly abuse survivors has completely

changed my outlook on aging. It's made me more aware of how I want to be treated when I'm older, and what we need to do as a society to get there." This awareness is leading many young adults to engage in what might be called 'preventive advocacy' – working to change systems and attitudes now to create better outcomes for the future.

The preparation for old age might seem like a distant concern for young adults, but engagement with elder care issues is prompting earlier and more thoughtful consideration of aging. Financial advisors report an uptick in younger clients seeking guidance on long-term care planning. There's also growing interest in age-friendly urban design among young architects and city planners, suggesting a more holistic approach to preparing for an aging society.

Some retirement homes are capitalizing on this interest by creating intergenerational programs. These initiatives go beyond typical volunteer activities, fostering meaningful relationships between residents

and young adults. One innovative program pairs retirement home residents with college students studying gerontology, creating mentorship opportunities that benefit both groups. The students gain practical insights into aging issues, while the residents enjoy the mental stimulation and social connection.

Yet, challenges remain in fully engaging young adults in elder abuse prevention. Time constraints, competing priorities, and the emotional weight of confronting abuse can be significant barriers. Additionally, some young adults may feel intimidated or unsure about how to effectively contribute to such a complex issue.

To address these challenges, many organizations are developing structured programs specifically designed for young adult involvement. These programs provide training, support, and clear pathways for engagement. They also emphasize the transferable skills that young adults can gain through their involvement – leadership, communication, empathy, and advocacy skills that are valuable in any career path.

The future of elder abuse prevention will likely depend significantly on the continued engagement of young adults. As this generation moves into positions of influence in healthcare, policy, and technology, their early experiences with elder care issues will inform their decisions and priorities. The seeds of change being planted today through youth engagement have the potential to grow into more comprehensive and effective approaches to preventing and addressing elder abuse.

As we look ahead, it's clear that young adults will play an increasingly vital role in shaping the future of elder care. Their energy, technological literacy, and fresh perspectives are invaluable assets in the fight against elder abuse. By fostering intergenerational connections and empowering young advocates, we can work towards a future where all seniors receive the care, respect, and dignity they deserve.

The engagement of young adults in elder abuse prevention represents more than just an additional resource – it symbolizes hope for a future where the vulnerability of age doesn't diminish the value of human dignity. As one young volunteer eloquently put it, "When we protect the dignity of our elders, we're really protecting the dignity of our future selves."

Preparation for Old Age

Perhaps the most profound impact of involving young adults in elder care is how it shapes their preparation for their own aging process. Through their experiences with elderly residents and exposure to the realities of retirement homes, young adults are beginning to think critically about their own future needs and the kind of elder care system they want to exist when they reach their senior years.

This forward-thinking approach is manifesting in several ways. Young adults are:

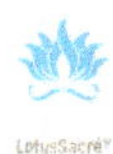

1. Starting to consider long-term care planning earlier in life
2. Showing increased interest in healthcare policies affecting the elderly
3. Becoming advocates for better retirement home conditions and regulations
4. Developing innovative technologies and solutions for elder care

Financial advisors report a growing trend of young clients seeking guidance on retirement planning and long-term care insurance, directly influenced by their experiences with elderly individuals in retirement homes. This early preparation extends beyond financial aspects to include considerations about healthcare preferences, living arrangements, and support systems.

The exposure to current retirement home conditions is also inspiring young adults to envision and work toward better alternatives for the future. Some are pursuing careers in fields where they can directly impact elder care, such as

healthcare administration, policy-making, or retirement home management. Others are exploring entrepreneurial ventures aimed at improving elder care through technology or innovative service models.

Young adults' preparation for old age is characterized by a more holistic approach than previous generations. Having witnessed both the challenges and possibilities in current retirement homes, they are better equipped to advocate for and work toward improvements in the system. This preparation extends to advocating for policy changes that will affect elder care in the decades to come.

Impact and Future Implications

The role of young adults in addressing elder abuse in retirement homes represents a significant shift in how our society approaches this critical issue. Their involvement brings fresh perspectives, energy, and innovative solutions to long-standing problems. As these young adults move into positions of influence in various

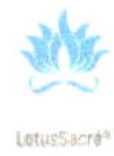
LotusSacré

sectors, their early experiences with elder care issues will inform their decisions and priorities.

The awareness, commitment, and forward-thinking preparation demonstrated by young adults today are laying the groundwork for better elder care in the future. Their role is not just about preventing abuse in current retirement homes, but about reshaping the entire paradigm of how we approach aging and elder care as a society.

As we look ahead, the continued engagement of young adults in this issue remains crucial. Their involvement not only benefits current elderly residents but also helps create a future where retirement homes are safer, more dignified, and better equipped to meet the needs of an aging population. By fostering this intergenerational approach to elder care, we move closer to a society where the vulnerability of age does not diminish the value of human dignity.

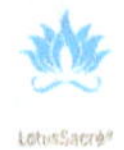

CALL TO ACTION

- If you're a young adult, volunteer at a retirement home.
- Start an intergenerational program in your community, connecting youth with elders.
- Create a social media campaign to raise awareness among young people about elder care issues.

Please Share Your Thoughts on Amazon!

Your Review Helps:

- Raise awareness about elder abuse in retirement homes
- Support independent authors tackling crucial social issues
- Encourage more research and action on elder care reform

How to Leave a Review:

- Go to the book's Amazon page
- Click "Write a customer review"
- Share your honest thoughts and experiences
- Click submit

If you found value in this book, please consider leaving a 5-star review!

Your support helps fuel further investigation into elder care issues and promotes positive change in our retirement homes. By sharing your thoughts, you're giving a voice to those who often go unheard and contributing to a movement for dignity and respect for our elders.

Together, we can make a difference in the lives of our seniors.

This version maintains the structure and purpose of the original text while adapting the content to fit the theme of your book on elder abuse in retirement homes. It emphasizes the importance of raising awareness about elder abuse and encourages readers to contribute to positive change through their reviews.

CHAPTER 9

FINANCING PROBLEMS FOR RETIREMENT HOMES IN FRANCE

The financial landscape of retirement homes in France is complex and increasingly problematic, presenting significant challenges for operators, residents, and the French healthcare system as a whole. As the population ages and demand for elderly care services grows, the financial sustainability of retirement homes has come under intense scrutiny. This chapter explores the multifaceted financial challenges facing French retirement homes, examining their causes, impacts, and potential solutions.

LotusSacré™

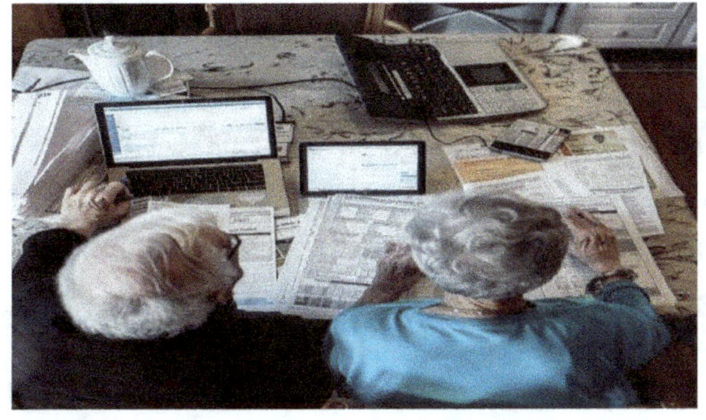

The Public-Private Divide: A System Under Strain

The French retirement home system operates on a unique model that combines public funding with private payments, creating a complex financial ecosystem. Public nursing homes, known as EHPAD (Établissement d'Hébergement pour Personnes Âgées Dépendantes), receive government subsidies but still require significant contributions from residents. Private facilities, both non-profit and for-profit, must balance their books while competing for clients and maintaining quality care.

The strain on this system has become increasingly evident. Public facilities

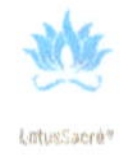

struggle with limited budgets that haven't kept pace with rising costs, while private homes face pressure to generate returns for investors without compromising care quality. This divide has created a two-tier system where the quality of care often correlates with a resident's ability to pay.

Adding to the complexity, the funding structure for French retirement homes involves multiple intertwined sources. Healthcare costs are covered by national health insurance, while dependency care is partially funded by the APA (Allocation Personnalisée d'Autonomie). Accommodation costs are primarily borne by residents or their families. This tripartite financing system, while designed to distribute costs fairly, has created administrative burdens and gaps in coverage. Many facilities find themselves caught between increasing regulatory requirements and insufficient funding to meet these standards.

Rising Costs vs. Limited Resources

The financial challenges facing French retirement homes are exacerbated by steadily rising costs across multiple fronts. Staffing represents the largest expense for most facilities, and these costs have increased due to various factors. Mandatory staffing ratios require more personnel, while higher wages are needed to attract and retain qualified caregivers. Additionally, increased training requirements and professional development costs put further strain on budgets.

Simultaneously, operational costs have surged dramatically. Energy and food prices have risen significantly, while medical supplies and equipment costs continue to climb. Regulatory compliance requirements demand ongoing investments, yet the resources available to retirement homes have not grown proportionally. Government funding, while significant, has failed to keep pace with these rising costs. The APA, intended to

help cover dependency care, often falls short of actual needs, leaving facilities and residents to make up the difference.

Private retirement homes have attempted to address this disparity by raising fees, but this approach has clear limitations. Higher fees can make care unaffordable for many seniors, creating occupancy challenges that further strain finances. Public facilities, constrained by regulations on what they can charge, often struggle to maintain quality standards with limited budgets.

The COVID-19 pandemic has intensified these financial pressures. Many homes incurred substantial additional expenses for protective equipment, testing, and extra staffing, while simultaneously experiencing reduced occupancy rates due to health concerns and temporary admission freezes. This perfect storm of increased costs and decreased revenue has pushed many facilities to their financial limits.

The Impact on Quality of Care and Potential Solutions

The financial constraints facing French retirement homes have direct implications for the quality of care they can provide. When budgets are tight, facilities often face difficult choices that impact various aspects of their operations. Staff numbers might be reduced, or less qualified personnel hired to cut costs. Non-essential services and activities often face cutbacks, while maintenance and upgrades to facilities may be deferred. Even daily aspects of care, such as meal options, can be affected as homes seek to reduce expenses.

These compromises significantly impact residents' quality of life and the overall standard of care. Moreover, financial pressures can create a stressful environment for staff, leading to higher turnover rates and potentially compromising care quality further. The ripple effects of financial constraints touch every aspect of retirement home operations.

However, various stakeholders are exploring potential solutions to these financial challenges. Some experts advocate for a complete overhaul of the current tripartite financing system. This could involve increasing the national insurance contribution to healthcare costs or expanding the APA to cover a larger portion of dependency care. Others propose creating a new national fund specifically for elderly care.

Private sector solutions are also emerging in response to these challenges. Some facilities are experimenting with social impact bonds to fund improvements in public facilities, while others explore cooperative models where residents become stakeholders. Partnerships between public and private entities to share resources and costs represent another innovative approach to addressing financial constraints.

Technology may also offer some relief from financial pressures. Investment in automation for administrative tasks could

reduce overhead costs, while telehealth services might provide more efficient medical care. Smart monitoring systems could help optimize staffing levels, allowing facilities to allocate their resources more effectively.

The French government has recognized the urgency of addressing these financial issues. Recent policy discussions have centered on potential reforms, including increased public funding for retirement homes and measures to make care more affordable for residents while ensuring facility sustainability. Some regions have undertaken local initiatives, experimenting with new funding models or providing additional support to struggling facilities. These localized approaches could provide valuable insights for broader national solutions.

The Deepening Financial Crisis in French Retirement Homes

The Hidden Cost of Care

Behind the polished facades of many French retirement homes lies a deepening financial crisis that threatens the very foundation of elderly care in France. The financial burden extends far beyond the visible costs of accommodation and basic care. Many families are shocked to discover the extensive array of additional charges that come with placing a loved one in a retirement home. These hidden costs often catch families unprepared, creating financial stress that ripples through generations.

Daily life in French retirement homes involves numerous expenses that aren't immediately apparent. Simple services that many assume would be included often come with additional fees. A resident might need to pay extra for services like accompanying them to medical appointments outside the facility,

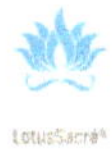

participating in certain activities, or even for basic hygiene products. These incremental costs add up quickly, turning what families thought would be a manageable expense into a significant financial burden.

The situation becomes even more complex when considering the geographical disparities in retirement home costs across France. In urban areas, particularly in and around Paris, the costs can be astronomical, forcing many families to look for options far from their homes. This geographical disparity creates a social equity issue, where access to quality care becomes increasingly dependent on a family's financial resources and location.

The Toll on Families

The financial strain of supporting a relative in a French retirement home often extends well beyond the elderly resident. Middle-aged children find themselves caught in a financial vice, simultaneously supporting their own children while contributing to

their parents' care costs. This "sandwich generation" faces difficult choices, sometimes delaying their own retirement or taking on debt to ensure their parents receive adequate care.

Some families resort to creative but potentially risky financial strategies to manage these costs. Children might take out second mortgages on their homes, liquidate savings intended for their own retirement, or even return to work after retirement themselves. The psychological impact of these financial pressures can be severe, creating tension within families and adding emotional stress to an already challenging situation.

Estate planning has become increasingly complicated as families try to navigate the financial implications of long-term care. Many elderly French citizens find themselves in the painful position of watching their life savings and intended inheritance diminish rapidly, leading to guilt and anxiety about becoming a burden on their children. This financial drain can

significantly impact intergenerational wealth transfer, affecting families' long-term financial stability.

The Market Forces at Play

The privatization trend in the French retirement home sector has introduced complex market dynamics that significantly impact financing. Large corporate groups have entered the market, bringing efficiency but also profit-driven approaches to elder care. These companies must balance shareholder expectations with the need to provide quality care, often leading to difficult compromises.

Real estate plays a crucial role in the financial equation of retirement homes. Many facilities operate under a model where they must generate returns not just from care services, but also from the property itself. This dual pressure can lead to situations where financial considerations overshadow care quality. Some operators focus on developing facilities in areas with high property values, potentially neglecting

regions where care is needed but less profitable.

The competition for qualified staff adds another layer to the financial challenges. Retirement homes must offer competitive salaries to attract and retain skilled caregivers, yet these increased labor costs often can't be fully passed on to residents without making the services unaffordable. This creates a constant tension between maintaining care quality and financial sustainability.

The Insurance Predicament

Long-term care insurance in France remains underdeveloped compared to some other countries, leaving a significant gap in financing options for elderly care. Private insurance products exist but often come with limitations and exclusions that make them inadequate for many people's needs. The premiums for comprehensive coverage are often prohibitively expensive, especially if purchased later in life.

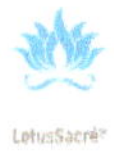

The French social security system, while robust in many areas, struggles to fully address the long-term care needs of an aging population. The existing benefits, such as the APA, were designed in a different era and haven't kept pace with the increasing costs and complexity of modern elder care. This gap between social coverage and actual costs creates a significant financial burden for many families.

Some innovative insurance products have emerged, attempting to bridge this gap. These include hybrid products that combine life insurance with long-term care benefits, or family-oriented policies that help distribute the financial risk among multiple family members. However, the uptake of these products remains limited, partly due to their complexity and partly due to a cultural reluctance to plan financially for potential dependency.

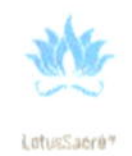

The Innovation Imperative

Financial innovations in the retirement home sector are emerging, though progress is slow. Some facilities are experimenting with flexible pricing models, where residents pay based on their actual use of services rather than a one-size-fits-all fee. Others are exploring community-based financing options, where local residents can invest in retirement homes, creating a sense of shared ownership and responsibility.

Technology is beginning to play a role in addressing some financial challenges. Automated systems for medication management, monitoring, and routine care tasks can help reduce staffing costs without compromising care quality. However, the initial investment required for these technologies can be substantial, creating another financial hurdle for many facilities.

Some retirement homes are diversifying their revenue streams by offering services to the broader community. This might

include operating day programs for seniors living at home, providing meals-on-wheels services, or renting out facilities for community events. While these initiatives can help support the financial bottom line, they also require careful management to ensure they don't detract from the core mission of resident care.

The Path Forward

As France grapples with these financial challenges, it's clear that a comprehensive rethinking of retirement home financing is needed. This might involve creating new financial products specifically designed for long-term care, developing more robust public-private partnerships, or fundamentally restructuring how care is funded and delivered.

The concept of intergenerational living is gaining traction as a potential partial solution to the financial crisis. Some innovative projects are exploring ways to combine student housing with retirement homes, creating mutually beneficial

arrangements that can help offset costs while fostering valuable social connections.

As the population continues to age, the financial sustainability of retirement homes in France remains a critical challenge that affects not just the elderly and their families, but society as a whole. Finding solutions will require creativity, collaboration, and a willingness to rethink traditional approaches to elder care financing.

The financial challenges facing French retirement homes are significant and complex, with no easy solutions in sight. The current system, stretched between public service obligations and financial sustainability, requires thoughtful reform to ensure quality care for France's aging population. As the country grapples with these issues, it's clear that any viable solution will require a multi-faceted approach, combining increased public funding, innovative financial models, and technological advancements. The stakes are high – the financial health of retirement

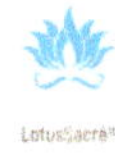
LotusSacré

homes directly impacts the quality of life for some of France's most vulnerable citizens.

Moving forward, the key will be finding a balance between financial sustainability and the fundamental mission of retirement homes: providing dignified, high-quality care for the elderly. As France continues to debate and develop solutions to these financial challenges, the experiences and lessons learned will likely provide valuable insights for other countries facing similar issues in their elderly care systems. The resolution of these financial difficulties will shape the future of elderly care in France and potentially serve as a model for addressing similar challenges worldwide.

CALL TO ACTION

- Engage in discussions about sustainable funding models for elder care.
- Write op-eds or start a blog to discuss innovative financing solutions for retirement homes.

- Organize a town hall meeting with local officials to discuss funding challenges and potential solutions.

Please Share Your Thoughts on Amazon!

Your Review Helps:

- Raise awareness about elder abuse in retirement homes
- Support independent authors tackling crucial social issues
- Encourage more research and action on elder care reform

How to Leave a Review:

- Go to the book's Amazon page
- Click "Write a customer review"
- Share your honest thoughts and experiences
- Click submit

If you found value in this book, please consider leaving a 5-star review!

Your support helps fuel further investigation into elder care issues and promotes positive change in our retirement

homes. By sharing your thoughts, you're giving a voice to those who often go unheard and contributing to a movement for dignity and respect for our elders.

Together, we can make a difference in the lives of our seniors.

This version maintains the structure and purpose of the original text while adapting the content to fit the theme of your book on elder abuse in retirement homes. It emphasizes the importance of raising awareness about elder abuse and encourages readers to contribute to positive change through their reviews.

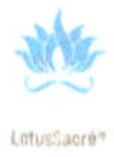

CONCLUSION

As we reach the end of our exploration into the deeply troubling issue of elder abuse in retirement homes, we are left with a profound sense of urgency and responsibility. The journey through the pages of this book has been challenging, often heartbreaking, but ultimately necessary. We have shed light on a crisis that has remained in the shadows for far too long, affecting some of the most vulnerable members of our society.

Reflecting on Our Journey

Our investigation began with a look at the history of retirement homes, tracing their evolution from charitable institutions to the complex, often profit-driven entities they are today. We've seen how the noble intention of providing care and dignity to our elders in their twilight years has, in many cases, been corrupted by systemic

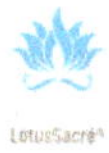

failures, financial pressures, and societal indifference.

The scandals we've uncovered and discussed are not isolated incidents but symptoms of a deeply rooted problem. From the shocking revelations in "Les Fossoyeurs" by Victor Castanet to the countless testimonies from victims and their families, we've seen a pattern of abuse that spans continents and cultures. These stories have forced us to confront an uncomfortable truth: our society has failed in its duty to protect and care for its elders.

We've delved into the various types of abuse - physical, psychological, neglect, and financial - each leaving its own devastating impact on the victims. The faces and stories behind these statistics remind us that each instance of abuse represents a human tragedy, a life diminished, and a family left in anguish.

Our examination of the contributing factors revealed a perfect storm of issues: understaffing, inadequate training,

financial pressures, and management failures. We've seen how the pursuit of profit can sometimes overshadow the core mission of care, leading to corner-cutting and neglect. But we've also recognized that many caregivers are themselves victims of a system that undervalues their work and stretches them to their limits.

The consequences of this abuse extend far beyond the immediate victims. We've explored how it impacts the physical and mental health of residents, the emotional toll on families, and the moral distress experienced by healthcare staff who find themselves unable to provide the level of care they know is needed.

Our international comparison showed us that while the problem is global, so too are the efforts to combat it. We've seen innovative approaches and reforms from countries around the world, proving that positive change is possible when there's political will and public engagement.

The Role of Society

Throughout this book, we've emphasized that elder abuse in retirement homes is not just a problem for the elderly or their immediate families - it's a societal issue that reflects on all of us. The way we treat our most vulnerable members speaks volumes about our values and priorities as a society.

Young adults, in particular, have a crucial role to play. Not only will they inherit the systems we create today, but they also have the energy, idealism, and technological savvy to drive significant change. We've discussed how increased awareness, volunteering, and preparing for their own old age can make a real difference.

The financial challenges facing retirement homes, particularly in countries like France, underscore the need for a broader societal conversation about how we fund and value elder care. It's clear that the current model is unsustainable and often incentivizes the wrong behaviors. We need innovative solutions that balance the need for quality care with financial sustainability.

Paths Forward

Despite the grim picture painted by much of our investigation, we've also found reason for hope. We've highlighted answers and solutions, from legislative reforms to grassroots initiatives, that are making a real difference in the lives of elderly residents.

Some key areas for improvement include:

1. **Enhanced Oversight and Accountability**: We need stronger regulatory frameworks with real teeth. This includes surprise inspections, clear reporting mechanisms for abuse, and significant penalties for facilities that fail to meet standards.

2. **Staff Support and Training**: Caregivers need better pay, manageable workloads, and comprehensive training. This

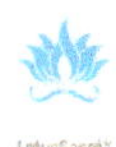

includes not just technical skills but also training in empathy, communication, and recognizing signs of abuse.

3. **Person-Centered Care Models**: We must move away from one-size-fits-all approaches to care. Instead, we should implement models that prioritize the individual needs, preferences, and dignity of each resident.

4. **Technology Integration**: While no substitute for human care, technology can play a crucial role in monitoring, safety, and enhancing quality of life for residents. From AI-powered abuse detection systems to communication platforms that keep families connected, tech solutions should be embraced and developed further.

5. **Community Integration**: Retirement homes shouldn't be islands unto themselves. We need to find ways to better integrate these facilities with the broader community, encouraging

LotusSacré™

intergenerational interactions and volunteering.

6. **Financial Reform**: We need to rethink how we fund elder care. This might involve new insurance models, public-private partnerships, or increased government funding. The goal should be a system that provides quality care without imposing crippling costs on families or incentivizing cost-cutting at the expense of care.

7. **Cultural Shift**: Ultimately, we need a fundamental shift in how society views and values its elderly members. This is a long-term project that involves education, media representation, and challenging our own biases about aging.

The Power of Individual Action

While the scale of the problem can seem overwhelming, it's crucial to remember that change often begins with individual actions. Throughout this book, we've provided calls to action at the end of each chapter,

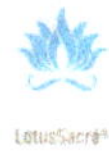

offering concrete steps that readers can take to make a difference.

These actions range from personal commitments to community initiatives:

- Educating ourselves and others about the signs of elder abuse
- Volunteering at local retirement homes
- Advocating for policy changes at local and national levels
- Supporting organizations that fight for elder rights
- Preparing for our own old age and having crucial conversations with our families
- Challenging ageist attitudes in our daily lives

Each of these actions, no matter how small it might seem, contributes to a larger movement for change. They help to break the silence surrounding elder abuse and create a culture of respect and care for our older citizens.

The Role of Artificial Intelligence

As we look to the future, it's clear that technology, particularly artificial intelligence, will play an increasingly important role in addressing elder abuse. We've explored how AI can be used to detect patterns of abuse, enhance training for caregivers, and even provide companionship for residents.

However, it's crucial that we approach these technological solutions with careful consideration of ethical implications. AI should be a tool to enhance human care, not replace it. We must ensure that in our rush to innovate, we don't lose sight of the fundamental human need for connection and compassion.

A Call for Continued Vigilance

As we conclude this exploration, it's important to recognize that the work is far from over. Elder abuse in retirement homes is a complex, multifaceted problem that will

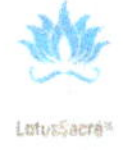

require ongoing attention, research, and action.

We must remain vigilant, continuing to shine a light on abuses where they occur and celebrating progress where we see it. This isn't just about protecting today's elderly population, but about creating a society that we ourselves would feel secure growing old in.

The Ripple Effect of Compassion

Every act of kindness, every policy change, every conversation about elder care sends ripples through our communities. By treating our elders with dignity and respect, we not only improve their lives but also set an example for future generations.

We're creating a legacy of compassion that will shape how we ourselves are treated in our later years. In this way, the fight against elder abuse is deeply personal for each of us, regardless of our current age.

Looking Ahead

As we close this book, let's envision a future where retirement homes are places of dignity, joy, and continued growth. A future where our elders are valued for their wisdom and experience, where caregivers are respected and supported in their crucial work, and where families can have peace of mind knowing their loved ones are in good hands.

This vision is within our reach, but it will take all of us - individuals, communities, institutions, and governments - working together to make it a reality. The stories and insights shared in this book are not the end of the conversation, but rather an invitation to deepen our commitment to this vital cause.

Your Role in Creating Change

As you finish reading this book, take a moment to reflect on what you've learned and how it has affected you. What actions are you inspired to take? How can you use

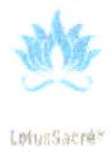

your unique skills, experiences, and position in your community to make a difference?

Remember, change doesn't always come in grand gestures. Sometimes it's as simple as spending time with an elderly neighbor, educating a friend about the realities of elder abuse, or writing a letter to your local representative. Every action, no matter how small, contributes to the larger movement for elder rights and dignity.

In the end, how we treat our elders is a reflection of our values as a society. It's a measure of our compassion, our respect for human dignity, and our understanding of the interconnectedness of all stages of life. By fighting against elder abuse and striving to create a world where all older adults can live with dignity and respect, we're not just improving the lives of our elders - we're elevating our entire society.

As you close this book, carry with you the stories you've read, the insights you've gained, and the urgency of this cause. Let

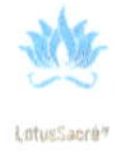

them inspire you to action, to conversation, and to a renewed commitment to creating a world where elder abuse is a thing of the past, and where growing old is a journey marked by dignity, respect, and joy.

The power to create this change lies with each of us. Together, we can build a future where every elder is valued, protected, and empowered to live their later years in peace and dignity. The journey starts now, with you.

www.ingramcontent.com/pod-product-compliance
Lightning Source LLC
Chambersburg PA
CBHW051601250726

48653CB00004BA/1268